The
Official Guide
to Medical School Admissions

How to Prepare for and Apply to Medical School

2015 Edition

The Official Guide to Medical School Admissions 2016–2017

AAMC Staff

MSAR® Program Staff
Tami Levin,
Director, MSAR and Aspiring Docs Programs

Nicole Lee,
Web & MSAR Content Specialist

Douglas Ortiz,
Director, Creative Services

Christina Scott,
Graphic Design Specialist

Content Specialist
Geoffrey Young, Ph.D.,
Senior Director,
Student Affairs and Programs

Consultants
Kelly Begatto,
Program Director, AMCAS®

Brent Bledsoe,
Senior Database Specialist

Lisa J. Jennings,
Senior Specialist,
Diversity Constituent Services

Jodi Lubetsky, Ph.D.,
Manager, Science Policy

David A. Matthew, Ph.D.,
Senior Research Analyst,
Student and Applicant Studies

H. Collins Mikesell,
Senior Research Analyst,
Student and Applicant Studies

Karen Mitchell,
Senior Director,
Admissions Testing Services

Julie Gilbert,
Senior Education Debt Management
Specialist

Jayme Bograd,
Director, Student Affairs

To order additional copies of this publication, please contact:

Association of American Medical Colleges
Publications Department
655 K Street, NW, Suite 100
Washington, DC 20001
Phone: 202-828-0416
email: *publications@aamc.org*
website: *www.aamc.org/publications*

Price: $15.00 for print edition,
plus shipping (single copy);
$15.00 for e-book/Kindle edition.

This is a publication of the Association of American Medical Colleges. The AAMC serves and leads the academic medicine community to improve the health of all.

The Official Guide to Medical School Admissions Kindle 2016–2017
978-1-57754-145-5

The Official Guide to Medical School Admissions e-book 2016–2017
978-1-57754-146-2

The Official Guide to Medical School Admissions 2016–2017
978-1-57754-148-6

Printed in the United States of America Revised annually; new edition available in early spring.

Group on Student Affairs (GSA) Steering Committee, 2014–2015

Chair
Robert L. Hernandez, M.D.
Associate Dean for Student Affairs
Florida International University Herbert
Wertheim College of Medicine

Chair Elect
Lee D. Jones, M.D.
Associate Dean for Student Affairs
University of California, Davis, School
of Medicine

Vice Chair
Thomas Koenig, M.D.
Associate Dean for Student Affairs
Johns Hopkins University School of Medicine

Immediate Past Chair
Marc J. Kahn, M.D., M.B.A.
Senior Associate Dean for Admissions &
Student Affairs
Tulane University School of Medicine

Previous Past Chair
W. Scott Schroth, M.D., M.P.H.
Associate Dean for Administration
George Washington University School of
Medicine & Health Sciences

Central Region Chair
Angela Nuzzarello, M.D., MHPE
Associate Dean for Student Affairs
Oakland University William Beaumont
School of Medicine

Northeast Region Chair
Carol A. Terregino, M.D.
Sr. Associate Dean for Education
Associate Dean for Admissions
Rutgers University – Robert Wood Johnson
Medical School

Southern Region Chair
Hilit F. Mechaber, M.D. q, FACP
Associate Dean for Student Services
University of Miami Miller School of Medicine

Western Region Chair
Donna Elliott, M.D., Ed.D., M.S.Ed.
Associate Dean for Student Affairs
Keck School of Medicine of the University of
Southern California

Chair, COA
Carolyn J. Kelly, M.D.
Associate Dean for Admissions and
Student Affairs
University of California, San Diego, School
of Medicine

Chair, COSDA
Wanda Lipscomb, Ph.D.
Senior Associate Dean of Diversity
and Inclusion
Associate Dean for Student Affairs
Michigan State University College of
Human Medicine

Chair, COSA
Anita Pokorny, M.Ed.
Director, Career Development and Advising
Northeast Ohio Medical University

Chair, COSFA
Cheri Marks
Coordinator, Financial Aid and
Student Records
University of Missouri-Columbia School
of Medicine

Chair, COSR
Rondel Frank, M.H.A.
Registrar
Tulane University School of Medicine

COD Liaison
Cynda Johnson, M.D., M.B.A.
Dean
Virginia Tech Carilion School of Medicine

Chair, OSR
Jessica Fried
Student
Geisel School of Medicine at Dartmouth

NAAHP Liaison
Julie Chanatry
Chief Health Professions Advisor
Colgate University

Association of American Medical Colleges

The Association of American Medical Colleges (AAMC) has as its purpose the advancement of medical education and the nation's health. In pursuing this purpose, the AAMC works with many national and international organizations, institutions, and individuals interested in strengthening the quality of medical education at all levels, searching for biomedical knowledge, and applying these tools to providing effective health care.

As an educational association representing members with similar purposes, the primary role of the AAMC is to assist those members by providing services at the national level that will facilitate the accomplishment of their missions. Such activities include collecting data and conducting studies on issues of major concern, evaluating the quality of educational programs through the accreditation process, providing consultation and technical assistance to institutions as needs are identified, synthesizing the opinions of an informed membership for consideration at the national level, and improving communication among those concerned with medical education and the nation's health. Other activities of the AAMC reflect the expressed concerns and priorities of the officers and governing bodies.

In addition to the activities listed above, the AAMC is responsible for the Medical College Admission Test® (MCAT®) and the American Medical College Application Service® (AMCAS®) and provides detailed admissions information to the medical schools and to undergraduate premedical advisors.

Important Notice

The information in this book is based on the most recent data provided by member medical schools prior to publication at the request of the Association of American Medical Colleges (AAMC).

This material has been edited and in some instances condensed to meet space limitations. In compiling this edition, the AAMC made every reasonable effort to ensure the accuracy and timeliness of the information, and, except where noted, the information was updated as of February 2014. All information contained herein, however, especially figures on tuition and expenses, is subject to change and is non-binding for medical schools listed and the AAMC. All medical schools listed in this edition, as with other educational institutions, are also subject to federal and state laws prohibiting discrimination on the basis of race, color, religion, sex, age, disability, or national origin. Such laws include Title VI of the Civil Rights Act of 1964, Title IX of the Education Amendments of 1972, Section 504 of the Rehabilitation Act of 1973, the Americans with Disabilities Act, and the Age Discrimination Act of 1975, as amended. For the most current and complete information regarding costs, official policies, procedures, and other matters, individual schools should be contacted.

In applying to U.S. or Canadian medical schools, applicants need not go through any commercial agencies. The AAMC does not endorse any organization or entity that purports to assist applicants to achieve admission to medical school other than undergraduate premedical advisors and medical school admissions officers.

AAMC Commitment to Diversity and Inclusion

AAMC's mission is to serve and lead the academic medicine community to improve the health of all. As the U.S. population ages, grows more diverse, and disparities in health care persist, the benefits of diversity and inclusion become critical to addressing the health of the nation. The AAMC's commitment to diversity and inclusion in medicine and biomedical research spans more than three decades demonstrated by ongoing leadership and engagement in activities starting as early as high school that promote diversity and inclusion through programs, advocacy and research. Information about AAMC initiatives is available at www.aamc.org/diversity.

Contents

Contents

Tables & Charts

Letter from Dr. Darrell Kirch

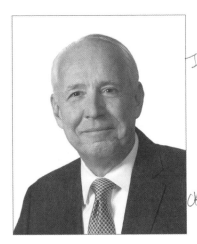

Maybe it was the great feeling you had from volunteering, or the profound concern stirred by a family member's illness that made you first think seriously about becoming a doctor. Or perhaps it was the thrill you experienced solving a complex research problem that inspired you to dream about finding the next "big cure." Whatever reason led you to consider a career in medicine, you have come to the right place: The Official Guide to Medical School Admissions.

Published annually by the Association of American Medical Colleges (AAMC)—the national association representing all 141 accredited U.S. and 17 accredited Canadian medical schools—the *Medical School Admission Requirements* guides are the only application resources authorized by medical schools themselves. The comprehensive *Medical School Admission Requirements* website will tell you about each school's focus, mission, and curriculum, as well as its entrance requirements and selection factors. *The Official Guide to Medical School Admissions* guidebook and e-book explain how medical schools increasingly are taking a holistic approach to admissions decisions by evaluating candidates' experiences and personal attributes in addition to their academic credentials and metrics, such as MCAT® exam scores.

On the *Medical School Admission Requirements* website, you will find details about financial aid and costs, and see the degree of diversity represented by 2014 matriculants. In what I think is one of the *Medical School Admission Requirements* website's best features, you will see that diversity reflected in the number of accepted applicants at each school who took certain premed courses, performed community service, or worked in research or other medically related positions. In other words, you will read about students who went through the same decision-making process you are undertaking now.

We have made a special effort to clarify the medical school application and admissions process. For example, the book provides a detailed description of the American Medical College Application Service® and a comprehensive look at the new MCAT2015, as well as a chapter on choosing the best school for you. We also have drawn from a wealth of data gathered by the AAMC and other sources to provide a more in-depth profile of today's medical students. For the first time this year, we have invited medical students to contribute essays introducing each chapter. You will read their personal perspectives on every step of the medical school application and admission process.

Should you decide to apply to medical school, I think you will find it is an extraordinary time to be a doctor. You will be entering medicine at a time when the country needs your services most, given predicted physician shortages in coming years, and when national attention is focused like never before on the need to improve health care delivery. Our profession is undergoing an exciting period of transformative change, with clinical care becoming increasingly patient-centered and team-based, biomedical research more technically sophisticated and collaborative, and medical education itself evolving into a continuum of lifelong learning.

Whatever career you decide to pursue, please accept my best wishes for success. If being a doctor is the path you choose, please know that the AAMC stands ready to help you. It would be a special pleasure for me if our paths should cross during your education and training and we have the opportunity to meet.

Darrell G. Kirch, M.D.
President and CEO, Association of American Medical Colleges

Letter from the Chair of the Organization of Student Representatives

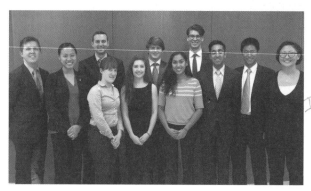

OSR Advisory Board 2015–16

Dear Medical School Applicant,

Congratulations on your pursuit of a career in medicine! You have embarked on a challenging but rewarding lifelong journey. In your future career as a physician, you will balance many roles to improve the health and well-being of the communities you serve, locally and abroad. You will develop and cultivate clinical skills and expertise to heal and comfort patients. You will be a lifelong learner and participate in the development of advanced technologies and treatment regimens. You will be an advocate, facilitator, and leader of interdisciplinary and interprofessional health care teams. You will touch the lives of your patients and their families; and at the same time, you too will be touched as you share in the very private and personal experience of illness.

The process of applying to medical school is overwhelming. Searching for the appropriate school that provides the opportunities you desire to meet your career goals is time-consuming, expensive, and challenging. To help demystify the process and guide you through the steps necessary to successfully complete the application process, the Association of American Medical Colleges (AAMC) has created this resource to help you along the way. The Medical School Admission Requirements guides will provide you with the most up-to-date information about U.S. and Canadian medical schools so that you can make a well-informed decision about how and where to pursue your medical studies.

As you navigate this process, you will find there is no one path to becoming a physician. Medical schools are searching for applicants with integrity, compassion, and altruistic ideals combined with a diverse set of experiences and backgrounds. Sir William Osler, a world-renowned physician, remarked to his students, "Live neither in the past nor in the future, but let each day absorb all your interest, energy, and enthusiasm. The best preparation for tomorrow is to live today superbly well." If your goal is to become a physician, stay focused, become as informed as possible, and persevere.

As chair of the AAMC Organization of Student Representatives (OSR), and on behalf of the 75,000 medical students and 110,000 resident physicians, we look forward to welcoming you into the profession as a future colleague. We hope you will join us as we commit ourselves to learn, serve, and lead in the health care of humanity.

Katie Maurer
5th year M.D./Ph.D. Student
New York University School of Medicine·
2014–2015 Chair
AAMC Organization of Student Representatives

Chapter 1:

So...You Want to Be a Doctor

Whether you witnessed a lifesaving moment, won the science fair, or volunteered in an under-resourced clinic, chances are something powerful influenced your decision to pursue the field of medicine.

Not everyone's journey to becoming a doctor is the same. Some students finish college and continue straight to medical school, others may work in another career first, some may choose to strengthen their skills and test their passion for medicine during a gap year. But if you have a passion for medicine, there is a path for you to get there.

In this chapter, you will read a synopsis of the steps involved and choices you will make as you pursue a medical career. Along the way, you will complete your undergraduate degree, take the Medical College Admission Test® (MCAT®), decide where to apply, navigate the application process, develop a financial strategy, and prepare for admission interviews. Big challenges lie ahead.

But so, too, does the ultimate reward: a career in medicine.

AAMC Official Information

Look for these icons throughout the Official Guide to get inside tips and information from the AAMC that you won't find anywhere else. This information comes from surveys of applicants, matriculants, medical students, graduates, and medical schools.

Tomorrow's Doctors, Tomorrow's Cures®

The dream of becoming a doctor is something that many of you knew from an early age. In fact, a recent AAMC survey shows that almost half of all entering medical students had decided upon a medical career before they set foot in undergraduate school—and one in five had made the decision before they even started high school.

Whether you have always known that you wanted to be a doctor, or are just starting to consider the idea, being a physician is an extremely rewarding profession. Nowhere else can you find a career that offers as many opportunities to make a real difference in the lives of countless people.

You will have job security knowing that your services will always be in demand. You will earn an excellent living. You will seldom experience the tedium of a nine-to-five desk job.

There is much more than that, though. As a doctor, you are likely to see new life come into the world or provide comfort to those about to leave it. Or you may choose to help build the future of medicine by educating the next generation of physicians. Perhaps you will dedicate yourself to discovering new cures for devastating diseases.

Whichever direction you follow, you will—either directly or indirectly—reduce or eliminate people's pain and suffering, improve their quality of life, and provide invaluable service to your local community or the country as a whole.

How many careers can even come close?

When Did You Decide to Study Medicine?

Most applicants knew early on that they wanted to be a doctor. According to an AAMC survey, half of all entering medical students made their decision to study medicine before they even started college:

- 19.7% before high school
- 30.6% during high school or before college
- 22.4% during first two years of college
- 10.3% during junior year of college
- 4.0% during senior year of college
- 10.7% after receiving bachelor's degree
- 2.3% after receiving advanced degree

Source: AAMC's 2014 Matriculating Student Questionnaire (MSQ)

What Specialties Are Entering Students Considering?

Medical students typically have clear preferences for the areas they plan to specialize in after graduation. However, many students change or further refine their specialty preferences as they gain experience and knowledge in medical school. The following list shows a breakdown of the percentage of students considering the specialties below.

Specialty	Percent
Internal Medicine	13.2
Pediatrics	11.2
Orthopedic Surgery	8.2
Emergency Medicine	8.0
Family Medicine	6.5
Obstetrics and Gynecology	4.3
Neurology	3.8
Radiology	1.7
Dermatology	2.5
Anesthesiology	2.1
Ophthalmology	1.9
Surgery	8.2
Neurological Surgery	2.3

Source: AAMC's 2014 Matriculating Student Questionnaire (MSQ)

Dozens of Options from Which to Choose

The fact that you have many options to choose from is another benefit of a career in medicine. From clinical practice to biomedical research, from public health to medical education—the choices are plentiful. If your interests change with time and experience, medicine—because of its emphasis on lifelong learning—will provide you with opportunities to refine your skills and reorient your practice. A number of possible career options are listed below:

- The satisfaction of long-term patient relationships is one attraction of **family medicine or internal medicine**, where the bulk of time is spent in direct contact with patients. Physicians who work under the umbrella of "primary care" often care for entire families and enjoy the challenges that come from treating a diverse population with varied backgrounds and conditions.

- Other physicians may prefer to pursue detailed knowledge about the intricacies of a single organ or system, such as that required of **cardiologists, ophthalmologists, dermatologists, and endocrinologists.**

- Interested in **scientific exploration** and the desire to **break new ground in medical knowledge?** Physicians with these interests are found in the nation's private and public laboratories and research institutions.

- Those with a commitment to social justice and an interest in fulfilling the health care needs of the underserved and disadvantaged can meet those challenges in **urban and rural clinics, public health, or as medical missionaries.**

- Careers in **general surgery** often suit those with a desire to see immediate results of their interventions. **Plastic and reconstructive surgery** draws others with artistic skills and aesthetic interests.

- Those interested in mind-body interactions and the emotional lives of their patients might find a home in **neurology or psychiatry.**

- The fast pace of medicine draws some to work as **emergency physicians or trauma surgeons.**

- Others motivated by the interest of national defense may use their skills as **flight surgeons or in military medicine.**

- The **economic and public policy aspects of health care** guide some physicians to think tanks and health-related organizations as well as serve in the legislative and executive branches of government.

- For those fascinated by the issues facing groups of patients with age-defined illnesses and problems—from the risks in infancy and early childhood to the challenges of older life—fulfillment can come in careers such as **pediatricians and geriatricians**.

- Assisting patients in overcoming complex fertility and gestational problems is the hallmark of the specialists in **reproductive endocrinology and obstetrics and gynecology.**

- Those dedicated to reducing the incidence of birth defects and inherited diseases might find their calling in **medical genetics.**

- The detection, prevention, and eradication of injury and disease draw people to the fields of **preventive medicine and epidemiology.**

Clearly, there are many possibilities in medicine. No matter what your personal interests, skills, or needs may be, medicine encourages you to find your niche.

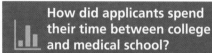

How to Decide Which Path Is "Best"

Which path is right for you? With the ever-changing world of medicine and a myriad of options and practice settings, figuring out where you belong as a physician can be one of the hardest decisions of your career.

Fortunately, you won't have to make this decision alone.

Medical schools realize how daunting this decision can be. They have a program in place to help you assess your personal values and interests, identify specialty options, determine personal "fit," and make a well-informed choice about your career path. The program, known as Careers in Medicine® (CiM), was developed by the AAMC in collaboration with its 141 member medical schools to guide you through the decision-making process.

The CiM program is completely free of charge for students attending AAMC-member medical schools. For more information, go to *www.aamc.org/cim*.

What About the Future?

As long as we are looking ahead, let's look way ahead. In five, 10, 15 years, what will medicine look like?

Recent Advances and Future Trends

One thing is certain—the face of medicine changes continually.* Take a look back just a single generation, and you will discover an abundance of fields that didn't exist.

- An obvious example dates back to the early 1980s. Back then, a new—and fatal—illness was taking hold that nobody could identify. We now know its name well—**AIDS**. Infectious disease is currently a large medical subspecialty and, as a result, significant advances have been made in extending the lives of those infected with HIV.

- Other advances are more recent. **Minimally invasive surgery**, in which surgeons carry out precise procedures with the assistance of a robot, is becoming increasingly popular. It is currently used for a variety of surgeries, including the lungs, esophagus, prostate, uterus, and kidneys. Through robotic-assisted surgery, patients are likely to benefit from smaller incisions, lower risk of complications, shorter hospital stays, less pain, and a speedier recovery.

- What about the advances in **personalized medicine**? A non-existent career path for the previous generation, the technology in this field allows physicians to identify mutated genes and alert patients of their predisposition to a specific disease. (The next step—actually treating disease with genes—is on the horizon.)

- Then there are more established fields that have evolved to take on new parameters. Take radiology, for example, which is no longer about just reading an X-ray. The radiologist can now perform the actual surgery as part of **interventional radiology**.

Even more exciting is what lies ahead: genetics therapy, portable medical records, distance surgery, and focused medication. The possibilities for advancement in medical research are limitless.

- Right now, physicians can diagnose predisposition to certain illnesses by identifying mutated genes. Currently in the research and development stage is the next step—**gene therapy**—in which physicians actually will replace defective genes by giving patients copies of the correct gene (which, in turn, "overtakes" the mutant gene).

* In the 1976–77 academic year, women comprised just 24.7 percent of all medical school matriculants. Compare that to 2014–2015, in which they made up almost half—or 47.8 percent—of the entering class. Source: AAMC Data Book.

Early tests have been especially favorable for cystic fibrosis, in which the correct CFTR gene is transported via a harmless virus or liposome.

- Similarly, research is underway in the field of **pharmacogenetics**—in which a patient's treatment is tailored according to the specific genetic code in question. For example, if a patient's genes fit a certain type of cancer code, the physician will prescribe the "matching" pharmaceutical that has been developed to destroy them—and will know, rather than hope, that the treatment is likely to work. Most forms of focused medication care involve oncology, but studies are progressing in areas of cardiology, diabetes, psychiatric disorders, and more.

- Also in development is **focused preventive care**, which, using genetic diagnosis, identifies to a very specific degree how likely a patient is to develop a certain disease or condition—and then prevents that development before it has a chance to begin.

- Other advances will be administrative in nature; the days of hunting down medical records may come to an end. One possibility being explored is a **portable medical records** system, or a national online database of individual health records. Everyone will carry a smart card (or have a microchip inserted under his or her skin!), allowing physicians to access medical records. The benefit? Errors are reduced, files can no longer be lost, delays are minimized, and the experience of having repeated—that is, unnecessary—tests is eliminated.

- And what about the robotics-assisted surgery we mentioned earlier? It provides the foundation for the next step forward—that of **distance surgery**. One day, surgeons will operate via a computerized system that will be located hundreds, even thousands of miles away from patients. This, of course, opens up a world of possibilities and opportunities in which specialists in one country can perform surgery on patients located in another.

Chart 1-A

Projected Supply and Demand, Physicians, 2008–2020

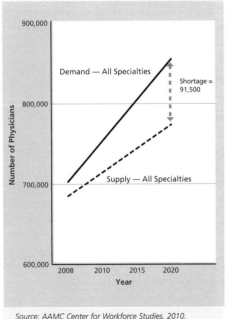

Source: AAMC Center for Workforce Studies, 2010.

Workforce Issues

Above all, know this: Whatever specialty you choose, your services as a physician will be needed.

According to the AAMC Center for Workforce Studies, there will be a shortage of 45,000 primary care physicians—and a shortage of 46,000 surgeons and medical specialists—in the next decade. The passage of health care reform, while setting in motion long-overdue efforts to insure an additional 32 million Americans, will increase the need for doctors and exacerbate a physician shortage driven by the rapid expansion of the number of Americans over age 65. Our doctors are getting older, too. Nearly one-third of all physicians will retire in the next decade just as more Americans need care. Continued demand for physicians and other medical professionals is obvious.

Chart 1-A illustrates the growing physician shortages between now and 2020. Still, the shortage will be experienced unevenly, and some areas will feel the effect more strongly than others. With that in mind, you may wish to consider the trends as you think about the direction you'd like your career to take.

Primary Care: Although the nation is facing an overall shortage of physicians, many are particularly concerned about the growing deficit of primary care doctors. To encourage more U.S. medical school graduates to pursue a career in primary care, the government is exploring ways to more fairly value primary care efforts and lessen administrative burdens associated with general medicine. You may want to explore the rewards this specialty offers, including the satisfaction that comes from delivering comprehensive care and the continuity of patient relationships.

FIN AID

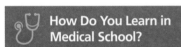
Underserved Areas: In addition, the impact of this shortage is expected to be greatest in underserved areas—the urban and rural areas where health care already is scarce. If you choose to serve in a community designated as a Health Professional Shortage Area, you may be able to take advantage of a federal program—the National Health Service Corps—which offers scholarships and loan repayment. *(Learn more about this program in Chapter 11: "You Can Afford Medical School.")*

A More Collaborative Approach — _Medical changes_ —

As Congress explores various scenarios as it moves toward instituting health care reform, one thing is all but certain: Given the projected shortage of physicians, we will need to develop new models of health care delivery that make better, more efficient use of all health care professionals—not just doctors. That means you can expect to work within a more collaborative, "shared" environment, in which a team of health care providers—including physician's assistants and nurse practitioners, for example—work more in tandem. Exactly how that will play out is still in the development stages, but the goal is to create a more efficient system, increase patient satisfaction, and, ultimately, improve health outcomes.

The Immediate Steps That Lie Ahead

That's the long-range future, or at least what we anticipate it is likely to entail. Right now, though, you're undoubtedly more focused on the short term—getting into medical school.

So what is the process like? What lies ahead?

Let's be candid. Getting into medical school isn't easy. (But it's definitely doable, a fact to which the more than 76,000 students currently there can testify!) You will need to prepare for and take the MCAT® exam, select appropriate schools to apply to, complete the application process, write a personal statement, gather letters of evaluation, and interview. And then you will wait for notices of acceptance and make your final decision. However, if you are not accepted, you will need to evaluate options and determine a course of action.

This will be covered in the following chapters.

But first, there are many steps you can take while still in college to make yourself a more attractive candidate to admissions committees. From taking the necessary courses, to working effectively with your pre-health advisor, to participating in extracurricular and volunteer activities that demonstrate your true interest in medicine, there's much you can do.

In the next chapter, we focus on your undergraduate preparation.

Chapter 2:
Building a Strong Foundation: Your Undergraduate Years

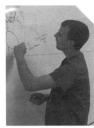

Matthew Rosenstein
M.D. Candidate
Duke University School
of Medicine
Class of 2018

Our paths to the M.D. degree begin well before we set foot on campus. For me, it started when my mom called me during my undergraduate freshman orientation. She encouraged me to take a chemistry class to prepare me for possibly applying to medical school. I remember asking, "But mom, do you really think I can get into medical school? It's so hard, and I don't really like the sight of blood, and I'm not good at biology." I signed up for that chemistry class, but my dream still seemed very distant until Dr. Isaac Yang, a neurosurgeon at UCLA, shared his journey with me. He didn't talk about grades, MCAT scores, or extracurricular activities. Instead, he shared his love for life and a life-changing experience when he saved a child from a traumatic brain injury on the streets of San Francisco. Years later, that same doctor who inspired me worked with me to co-edit a book of memoirs titled, The Service Minded Physician, *which is about how physician-leaders, including NIH Director Francis Collins, M.D., Ph.D. and AAMC President and CEO Darrell G. Kirch, M.D., have maintained their humanism.*

It's so easy to view the journey to medical school as a contest, but as I learned, it's much more about people than numbers. Think about why you're really reading this book, the kind of person you want to be beneath your white coat, and go change the world. In this chapter, you will learn about how to build a strong foundation during your undergraduate years. I'll see you on rounds in a couple years.

Academic Preparation

College coursework plays a major role in your preparation for medical school. Your academic groundwork and development includes your major field of study, the mastery of specific scientific principles, and advanced coursework. Let's take a look at each of these a bit further.

Choice of Major

Contrary to what many college students believe, there is no such thing as the "best" major. **In fact, no medical school requires a specific major of its applicants.** That's because admissions committee members know that students develop the essential skills of acquiring and synthesizing information through a wide variety of academic disciplines and, therefore, should be free to select whichever major they find interesting and challenging.

Even so, many premedical students choose to major in a scientific discipline. If that's the direction you're heading, and you're doing so because you are fascinated by science and believe that such a major will be the foundation for a variety of career options, great. If you're doing so because you believe it will enhance your chances for admission, think again.

How Do Students Prepare for Medical School?

College students take advantage of a variety of programs to prepare for medical school and a career in medicine. The following shows the percentage of students who participated in:

Program	Percent
Volunteered or worked in the health care field	91.5
MCAT® preparation course (university-based or private)*	59.6
Laboratory research apprenticeship	58.6
Summer academic enrichment	14.8
Postbaccalaureate program to complete premedical requirements	10.1
Postbaccalaureate program to strengthen academic skills	7.5

*This figure is comprised of all preparation programs, including no or low-cost university-provided preparation courses.
Source: AAMC's 2014 Matriculating Student Questionnaire (MSQ)

Table 2-A

Subjects Required or Recommended by 10 or More U.S. Medical Schools

Required/Recommended Subject	# of Schools
Behavioral Sciences	13
Biochemistry	41
Biology	94
Biology/Zoology	27
Calculus	12
College Mathematics	37
English	79
Humanities	15
Inorganic Chemistry	111
Organic Chemistry	115
Physics	111
Social Sciences	15

N=141. Some medical schools use a "competency" model that recommends competencies rather than specific coursework. For premedical coursework required by the specific medical schools in which you are interested, please see the Medical School Admission Requirements website (www.aamc.org/msar). Source: AAMC Medical School Admission Requirements website, 2015

Admissions committees welcome students whose intellectual curiosity leads them to a wide variety of disciplines.

And no…you won't be at a disadvantage if you choose to major in English, for example, rather than biology. Using just one measure, that of MCAT® scores, you may be surprised to learn that there is very little difference in median total scores among those who major in the humanities, social sciences, and biological sciences.

The Official Guide to the MCAT® Exam, a guidebook available for purchase at *www.aamc.org/officialmcatguide*, includes a chart that provides the median MCAT scores of applicants by undergraduate major. There you will see that the total median score for humanities, biology, and social sciences majors were 30, 28, and 29, respectively. This attests to the fact that students from any major, as long as they have the basic science preparation, are equally prepared for acceptance into medical school.

Scientific Preparation

Still, medical schools recognize the importance of a strong foundation in mathematics and the natural sciences—biology, chemistry, and physics— and most schools have established minimum course requirements for admission. These courses usually represent about one-third of the credit hours needed for degree completion (leaving room for applicants to pursue a broad spectrum of college majors, as mentioned on the left). In particular, medical schools expect that their entering students will have mastered basic scientific principles by successfully completing one academic year (two semesters or three quarters) of biology and physics and one academic year of general chemistry and one year of organic chemistry, including adequate laboratory experiences. Increasingly, biochemistry is strongly recommended by schools.

While only a few medical schools require applicants to complete a specific course in mathematics, all schools appreciate that mathematical competence provides a strong foundation for understanding basic sciences. A working knowledge of statistics helps students fully grasp medical literature, and familiarity with computers is valuable as well. Many medical schools therefore recommend coursework in mathematics and statistics in addition to the science courses named above. The table to the left gives an overview of the most common courses required by medical schools.

AP, IB, and CLEP Courses

Students who intend to apply college credit earned through **advanced placement (AP), international baccalaureate (IB), and college-level examination placement (CLEP)** to meet premedical requirements should be aware that some medical schools have requirements involving the use of such credit. Please review the *Medical School Admission Requirements* website (*www.aamc.org/msar*) and the websites of medical schools you're interested in for more information.

Competencies vs. Courses

Finally, for those of you reading this in the early years of college (or in high school), we would like to draw your attention to the fact that medical schools are increasingly defining their prerequisites by competencies—rather than courses. This comes about because, as a study undertaken by the Howard Hughes Medical Institute (HHMI) and the AAMC points out, the scientific knowledge medical schools seek in their applicants can be obtained in a variety of courses as opposed to specific ones. (In other words, a student might be able to master chemistry principles in a zoology class or statistics in a sociology course.)

Advanced Coursework

Although upper-level science coursework may not be required by every medical school, it is usually a good idea to show that you have challenged yourself academically. Successfully completing advanced courses demonstrates science proficiencies and ultimately strengthens your preparation for medical school. Taking science courses that simply duplicate basic content, however, is not recommended. But don't think that all of your courses must be STEM-based (science, technology, engineering, and math). Practicing physicians often suggest that premedical students take advantage of what might be their final opportunity for study in nonscience areas and take elective courses in subjects of interest such as music, art, history, and literature. Medical schools also are looking for applicants with rich and varied coursework and experiences. Beyond that, medical schools encourage honors courses, independent study, and research work by premedical students. Activities such as these demonstrate in-depth scholarly exploration and the presence of lifelong learning skills that are essential to a career in medicine.

Into the Future: Competency-Based Prerequisites

The Scientific Foundations for Future Physicians report (conducted by the AAMC-HHMI Scientific Foundation for Future Physicians committee) proposes scientific competencies for future medical school graduates and undergraduate students who want to pursue a career in medicine. Competencies entering medical students should demonstrate include:

- Both the knowledge of and ability to apply basic principles of mathematics and statistics, physics, chemistry, biochemistry, and biology to human health and disease

- The ability to demonstrate observational and analytical skills

- The ability to apply those skills and principles to biological situations

 You can download a free copy of this report at *www.aamc.org/scientificfoundations*.

Personal Attributes

 Academic and scientific accomplishments alone are not sufficient for a student to be accepted into medical school. While intellectual capacity is obviously important to be a successful physician, so are other attributes that signify the ability to develop and maintain effective relationships with patients, work collaboratively with other team members, act ethically and compassionately, and in many other ways master the "art" of medicine.

An AAMC publication titled *Learning Objectives for Medical Student Education: Guidelines for Medical Schools* (*www.aamc.org/initiatives/msop*) describes the personal attributes required of a physician. While making note of the fact that graduating medical students must be knowledgeable about medicine and skillful in its application, the publication also emphasizes how vital it is for students to:

- Make ethical decisions

- Act with compassion, respect, honesty, and integrity

- Work collaboratively with team members

- Advocate on behalf of one's patients

- Be sensitive to potential conflicts of interest

- Be able to recognize one's own limits

- Be dedicated to continuously improving one's knowledge and abilities

- Appreciate the complex nonbiological determinants of poor health

- Be aware of community and public health issues

- Be able to identify risk factors for disease

- Be committed to early identification and treatment of diseases

- Accept responsibility for making scientifically based medical decisions

- Be willing to advocate for the care of the underserved

Chances are, some of the most valuable traits you will demonstrate as a physician are not going to be learned in a classroom. These characteristics may be nurtured throughout your college years (and, as you will see in Chapter 7, are among the attributes that admissions officers seek when admitting applicants to their programs). You don't need formal programs to learn how to be a kind, empathetic physician. You will have an abundance of opportunities to develop these qualities through your interactions with friends, classmates, and others while in college and through your work experiences.

Extracurricular Activities Related to Medicine

Your undergraduate years offer opportunities to become involved in a wide range of extracurricular activities. Ideally, at least a few of them should involve the medical field. Experience in a health care setting; volunteering at shelters, clinics, or in other environments to care for ill or elderly people in your community; participating in basic or clinical research efforts; working as an emergency medical technician; "shadowing" a physician; providing support to people in a rape crisis center, emergency room, or social service agency—are types of activities recommended to those considering a career in medicine.

These pursuits provide you with the chance to learn more about the medical profession—and yourself. You will, for example, be able to:

- Explore different interests

- Test out your natural inclinations to one or more endeavors

- Better understand the nature of medical practice and the daily demands placed upon physicians

- Assess your ability to communicate and empathize with people from different backgrounds and cultures

- Evaluate your willingness to put others' needs before your own

While this self-analysis can help you decide if a career in medicine is right for you, your involvement with clinical or research activities helps demonstrate to admissions committees where your interests lie. It also shows that you have explored various aspects of the medical field. Admissions committees evaluate your experiences using at least three different criteria, and a greater value is assigned to certain types of pursuits than others.

Specifically, admissions committees look at the length of time you've invested, the depth of the experience, and lessons learned—in relation to any particular activity. This means a single daylong blood drive or one-time-only shadowing experience is less enlightening than semester or yearlong commitments. By the same token, active participation in an activity is viewed as more instructive than a passive one (such as observation). Most important, admissions committees want to know what students learned from their experiences, and you should therefore be prepared to address these kinds of questions about your community, clinical, or research experiences in your application materials (which will be discussed in Chapter 6: *Applying to Medical School*).

Pre-Health Advisors

Fortunately, you are not on your own when it comes to preparing for medical school. You have valuable resources available to you—some of which are likely available right on campus such as your pre-health advisor.

Depending on the individual school, pre-health advisors work on a full- or part-time basis, and may be faculty members (often in the science department), staff members in the office of an academic dean or in the career center, directors of an advising office for pre-professional students, or a physician in part-time practice. Advisors belong to organizations such as the National Association of Advisors for the Health Professions (NAAHP, *www.naahp.org*) that assist them in their work—and help them help you. If your school does not have a pre-health advisor available to you, the NAAHP has members who volunteer to help students who do not have access to an advisor. Visit *http://www.naahp.org/StudentResources/FindanAdvisor.aspx* for more information. You can always reach out to medical school admissions staff if you have specific questions about admission requirements or policies. Be sure to first check the medical school's website to see if the information is available.

Services Provided

The support provided by pre-health advisors varies according to a number of factors. Generally speaking, services fall into five categories:

- **Academics.** Advisors are well-informed about premedical coursework on their campuses and developing suitable academic programs for premedical students. They collaborate with campus academic staff in designing study, reading skills, and test-preparation workshops, offering tutoring programs, as well as informing their students of regional and national programs likely to be of interest.

- **Clinical and research experiences.** In working with advisory groups composed of college and medical school teaching and research faculty and community clinicians, advisors help identify part-time jobs, volunteer positions, and opportunities for independent study credit in local laboratories and offices.

- **Advising and support.** Advisors help students pursue realistic goals and maximize their potential, both meeting with them individually and providing group opportunities for students to meet with one another. Advisors often establish peer advising and mentoring programs and are particularly sensitive to the needs of students who are underrepresented in medicine or are the first in their family to attend college.

- **Assistance to student organizations.** Advisors coordinate the activities of local and national organizations that serve premed students by planning programs, identifying funding sources, and arranging for campus visits from admissions and financial aid officers.

- **Sharing resources.** Being aware of students' need for timely and pertinent information, advisors disseminate publications and other resources from relevant organizations, including the AAMC and NAAHP. In addition, advisors provide computer access to Web-based content on health careers programs and educational financing; distribute information about local, regional, national, and international research and service opportunities; and stock a library of publications related to medical school and medical education.

Contact your school's advisor to discuss the availability of these services.

The Pre-Health Committee Letter of Evaluation

There is another vital service that pre-health advisors offer their students (and often their alumni): the pre-health committee letter of evaluation.

This is usually a composite letter written on behalf of a medical school applicant by the college or university's pre-health committee. It presents an overview of the student's academic strengths, exposure to health care and medical research environments, contributions to the campus and community, and personal attributes such as maturity and altruism. In addition, the letter may address any extenuating circumstances that may have resulted in deficits in the student's performance during a course or semester, provide perspective on challenges the student may have encountered, and explain school-specific courses and programs in which the student has participated.

Some undergraduate institutions do not provide composite letters of evaluation but instead collect individual letters throughout the student's enrollment. Then, at the appropriate time, they distribute the letters to the medical schools where the student has applied.

Pre-Health Advisors: A Wide Range of Guidance

There are many instances in which a pre-health advisor may assist you, including:

- Identifying courses that satisfy premedical requirements

- Determining a sequence for completing those courses

- Finding tutorial assistance, if needed

- Planning academic schedules to accommodate both premedical coursework and other educational objectives, such as a study program abroad, a dual major, or a senior honors thesis

- Locating volunteer or paid clinical and research experience

- Strengthening your medical school application

- Preparing for interviews and standardized tests

- Arranging for letters of evaluation

- Determining the most appropriate career paths based on individual strengths, values, and life goals

Special Programs

Finally, we would like to draw your attention to the following two programs that may be of interest (depending on where you fall in the education process):

- **Combined Baccalaureate/M.D. Programs**
  If you're reading this book during the latter stages of high school, you might want to explore a combined B.S./M.D. program, offered at about a quarter of U.S. medical schools. Graduates of these programs, which range in length from six to nine years, receive both a bachelor's degree from the undergraduate institution and an M.D. from the medical school. For more details and a list of participating schools, please see Chapter 12 as well as the individual Baccalaureate/M.D. program profiles in the *Medical School Admission Requirements* website (*www.aamc.org/msar*).

- **Postbaccalaureate Programs**
  Perhaps you're at a different stage along the educational continuum and have already graduated from college. If your major was something other than science, it's

quite possible that you will need to pursue additional coursework before applying to medical school. Postbaccalaureate programs offered at colleges and universities across the country range from formal one- or two-year master's degree programs to certificate programs. These programs are available to help applicants who may need to strengthen their knowledge in the sciences, complete required premedical coursework, career chargers, or need academic enhancement. A searchable database of these programs can be found at *http://services.aamc.org/postbac*. You can also locate medical schools that have postbaccalaureate programs using the search features in the *Medical School Admission Requirements* website (*www.aamc.org/msar*).

Chapter 3:
Your Medical School Years:
The Education Process

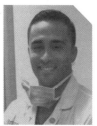

Edwin Acevedo, Jr.
M.D. Candidate
Robert Wood Johnson
Medical School
Class of 2015

Medicine is a lifelong commitment. Every medical student knows they must be ready to fully dedicate themselves to studying and adapting to the changes. But what does it really take to become a doctor?

The short answer is four years of medical school, a three- to eight-year residency program, and passing scores on three USMLE Step exams administered along the way. Truthfully, the medical education process is always evolving. Teaching methods, topics of interest, and technological innovations all will play a role in how you learn.

People often say that the volume of information you will learn in medical school is like "drinking from a fire hose." As a med student, you will change the way you learn, and you will adopt new study skills. You may study differently with every new step in the process of becoming a physician. You will go from rapidly absorbing a plate full of books in the preclinical years, to feeling like a hunter-gatherer learning on the go during clinical rounds with barely enough time to digest information.

And just when you think you've got it figured all out, you will learn in residency that every patient is different—there is no golden script. But yet, all of the information you gather is applicable in a different way for each patient.

The medical education process is vigorous, but it is this very process that makes medicine so beautiful. Here, we will cover how medical education has changed over time, what material you can expect to learn, and an overview of what you will be doing along the way.

Straight to Medical School from College...or a Gap Year First?

If a year or more has passed since you graduated from college, you are not alone. More than half of matriculating medical students—58.0 percent—indicated in a recent AAMC survey that there was a "gap" between college and medical school of at least a year.

Source: AAMC's 2014 Matriculating Student Questionnaire (MSQ)

Undergraduate Medical Education: An Overview of the Medical School Years

At the core, all U.S. and Canadian medical schools have the same purpose—to educate their students in the art and science of medicine, provide them with clinical experience, and, ultimately, prepare them to enter a residency program (also referred to as "graduate medical education"). That is why every school follows the same basic program—requiring students to acquire a basic foundation in the medical sciences, apply this knowledge to diseases and treatments, and master clinical skills through a series of "rotations."

That doesn't mean that a medical school...is a medical school...is a medical school. Far from it. Each school establishes its own curriculum and course format, so that, for example, a particular class required by one institution is an elective course in another. Even when medical schools seem to require identical courses, the content within them may differ, so that some of the material covered in immunology in one school, for instance, is presented in pathology in another. (The sequence in which courses are taken—and the method by which the content is taught—may differ, as well.) Beyond that, the processes by which students are graded also vary from school to school, with some institutions following a pass/fail system, others an honors/pass/fail system, and still others a letter grading system.

Medical schools must meet very exacting standards to earn (and maintain) accreditation, as established by the Liaison Committee on Medical Education (LCME). The LCME (*www.lcme.org*), cosponsored* by the AAMC and the American Medical Association, accredits medical school programs that grant the M.D. degree in the United States and reviews and approves curricula, organization, and student performance.

Beyond accreditation requirements, there are other strong parallels among medical schools' curricula. The general structure of the overall educational programs follow a similar path although there is significant overlap between what has traditionally been referred to as "preclinical" and "clinical" years.

A Word About Preclinical vs. Clinical Years

Medical school is commonly structured into two halves: preclinical years and clinical years.

Students typically concentrate their efforts on the scientific underpinnings of medicine during the first two years, and apply and refine that knowledge during a series of rotations during the second two years. However, there is often an overlap in content between these two stages of medical education. It is increasingly common for a student to have some clinical exposure in the first year of medical school. Similarly, during the clinical years, students refine their understanding of underlying medical concepts and apply basic science knowledge. It is important, therefore, to recognize that preclinical and clinical content can—and does—intersect at any stage in the medical school experience.

Building a Foundation of Knowledge

In almost all cases, you'll begin your medical school studies by learning how the human body is supposed to work—both in terms of structure and function. The focus will then shift to abnormal conditions and diseases, methods of diagnosis, and treatment options.

- **Normal Structure and Function**
  Before learning about illnesses and ailments, one of the first important concepts is to understand how the healthy body works. How does the healthy body work? That's what you'll be studying right out of the starting gate, and your courses will be many—and varied. Typically, your basic classes will include gross and microscopic anatomy, physiology, biochemistry, behavioral sciences, and neurology.

- **Abnormalities, Diagnostics, and Treatment**
  After you have learned what "healthy" looks like (and acts like), the focus of your coursework will shift again, in terms of both structure and function. You will study the full range of diseases and atypical conditions, methods by which diagnoses are made, and therapeutic principles and treatments. It is at this stage that you'll have classes in immunology, pathology, and pharmacology.

*Accreditation by the LCME is required for schools to receive federal grants and to participate in federal loan programs. In addition, eligibility of U.S. students to take the United States Medical Licensing Exam (USMLE)—a discussion of which appears in "Licensure and Certification: Ready to Function Independently" later in this chapter—requires LCME accreditation of their school. All medical schools listed in this guide are accredited by the LCME.

- *Other Topics*

    You will be exposed to a wide variety of other topics. These will range from nutrition, to medical ethics, to genetics…from laboratory medicine, to substance abuse, to geriatrics. Health care delivery systems. Human values. Research. Preventive medicine. Human sexuality. Community health. The fact is that the subjects taught at medical schools are as varied, and potentially as numerous, as are the institutions themselves.

And that's just part of the picture. There's much more to "building a foundation" than mastering the scientific basis of medicine. During this period of your medical education, you will learn the basics of taking patient history, conducting physical exams, interpreting laboratory findings, and considering diagnostic treatment and alternatives—in effect, readying yourself for the clinical rotations that follow in the latter half of medical school.

Finally, keep in mind that practicing medicine is not all science—or even the application of science (such as that required to interpret lab results and figure out a course of treatment). Medical schools recognize that physicians practice in a social environment—one in which effective team building, collaboration, and communication skills are necessary. As a result, the very way in which students learn and are taught has evolved in recent years. (This is discussed in more depth on the next page—"Changing Face of Medical Education.")

Acquiring Hands-On Experience Through Clerkships

A major component of your undergraduate medical education, typically during the third and fourth years, will be a series of required clinical clerkships or "rotations." Under direct supervision of a faculty member and/or resident, each clerkship can range from four to 12 weeks and provides students with firsthand experience working with patients and their families and in inpatient and outpatient settings.

While the pattern, length, and number of rotations differ from school to school, core clinical training usually includes clerkships in internal medicine, family medicine, obstetrics/gynecology, pediatrics, psychiatry, and surgery. Beyond that, and depending on your specific school's requirements, your program also may include clerkships in primary care and neurology, for example, or require participation in a community or rural program.

- *What You'll Do*

    During a clerkship, you'll be assigned to an outpatient clinic or inpatient hospital unit where you will assume responsibility for "working-up" a number of patients each week—collecting relevant data and information from them—and presenting findings to a faculty member. Beyond that, you'll participate in the ongoing care of patients, either during hospitalizations or through the course of outpatient treatment, and, when appropriate, interact not only with the patients themselves, but also with their families.

- *And What You'll Learn*

    There's no substitute for "hands-on" experience—and plenty of it. During the course of your clerkships, you'll learn to apply basic science knowledge and clinical skills in diagnosing and treating patients' illnesses and injuries and will become adept at interacting with patients (and their families) as you provide information, answer questions, and prepare them for the likely outcome. At the same time, you'll become effective working with all members of the health care team, whether at the bedside, during inpatient team discussions ("rounds"), or in case-based lectures and small group discussions.

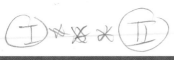

What A Typical Curriculum* May Include

Year 1 – Normal structure and function
Biochemistry, cell biology, medical genetics, gross anatomy, structure and function of human organs, behavioral science, and neuroscience

Year 2 – Abnormal structure and function
Abnormalities of structure and function, disease, microbiology, immunology, pathology, and pharmacology

Years 3 and 4 – Clinical clerkships
Generalist core: family and community medicine, general and ambulatory care, internal medicine, obstetrics and gynecology, pediatrics, surgery, and research

Other requirements: neurology, psychiatry, subspecialty segments (anesthesia, dermatology, urology, radiology, etc.), emergency room and intensive care experiences, and electives

*The curriculum outlined above is a representation only—and not inclusive of all courses/clerkships.

Electives

Just like college, you'll enjoy an opportunity to explore special interests by way of electives. Offered in basic, behavioral, and clinical sciences, as well as in basic and clinical research, electives usually are available during your final year of medical school (although you might be able to take them at other times). They may be completed on your own campus, at other medical schools through a "visiting student program," through federal and state agencies, in international settings, and service organizations.

The Changing Face of Medical Education

Some of you may have heard of Abraham Flexner, who wrote a groundbreaking report on medical education in 1910. Although the basics of his model have survived to the present day—mainly, a four-year program affiliated with a university*—he never intended it to serve for more than a generation. After all, no one can predict the future.

Time has certainly proven him correct.

There is no way that Flexner could have anticipated the shifting demographics, technological advances, and evolving teaching techniques of the late 20th century and the first decade of the 21st century. You, on the other hand, will experience firsthand the reforms taking place in medical education—both in terms of what you'll learn and how you'll learn it. Your courses may range from cultural competency to health care financing, and you'll benefit from educational developments such as computer-aided instruction, virtual patients, and human patient simulation. It's an exciting time to be a medical student.

What You'll Learn

You are going to have to wield a scalpel in anatomy class early on in medical school, just as students in our parents' and grandparents' generations did 30 and 60 years ago. Certain things stay the same. That type of effort aside though, there are many significant changes in medical education content, and schools are continually revising their curricula to reflect advances in science, breakthroughs in medicine, and changes in society. For example:

- Consider the demographic shift we will experience as the baby boomers age. By 2030, the population of those over age 65 is expected to double, and physicians will spend an increasing amount of time treating age-related problems such as Alzheimer's, heart failure, pulmonary disease, and bone disorders. As a result, most medical schools now include in their curricula courses on geriatrics, palliative care, pain management, complementary medicine, and other similar age-based material.

- Issues such as health literacy, nutrition, drug abuse, and domestic violence are important components of medical education. Because many of these and other health problems are related to culture and lifestyle, medical schools have increasingly focused efforts on areas such as disease prevention, health promotion, population health, and cultural diversity.

- Medical schools are placing an increasingly important emphasis on helping their students develop effective communication skills, allowing them to interact successfully with a diverse group of patients. You'll be directly taught to assess family, lifestyle, and socioeconomic factors that may influence your patients' behavior, or affect their care.

Then, of course, there are the advancements in science and medicine themselves. (As researchers make breakthroughs in genetic diagnoses and treatments, for instance, that new knowledge is incorporated into the medical school program.) There are also expanded

*At the time of Flexner's report, many medical schools were small trade schools unaffiliated with a university, and a degree was awarded after only two years of study.

Changing Demographics = Changing Education

The U.S. population over age 65 is expected to be almost 70 million by 2030—accounting for one in every five Americans. Demographics such as that, together with advanced technologies, scientific discoveries, and evolving teaching techniques, all contribute to significant changes in medical education.

Source: Population Projections of the U.S. by Age, Sex, Race and Hispanic Origin: 1995-2050, US Bureau of the Census.

Examples of "New" Topics in Medical Education

Of 140 medical schools surveyed, the following topics were required at the vast majority of institutions:

Topic Area	# of Medical Schools Requiring Topic
Cultural Competence	139
Substance Abuse	137
Communication Skills	138
Preventive/Health Maintenance	136
Medical Genetics	140
Domestic Violence/Abuse	138
Pain Management	137
Health Care Systems	134
Complementary/Alternative Health Care	126
Health Care Financing	123

Source: 2013–2014 LCME Part II Annual Medical School Questionnaire

courses on medical ethics, examining some of the dilemmas physicians may face amid the advent of new technology; classes on financial decision making, in which students are taught to weigh the likely costs and benefits of various treatments; and sessions on evidence-based medicine and patient quality, providing students with the information and tools they will need to deliver the best possible care.

The topics described here are only an overview of some possibilities. The specific courses you'll take as a medical student will vary depending on the school.

How You'll Learn It

Do you have an image of sitting in a large lecture hall, surrounded by hundreds of your peers? While you'll certainly experience that aspect of medical school, that method of teaching is being replaced (to a significant degree) by other techniques. Here are a few of the most widespread methods:

- The traditional lecture-based approach is increasingly giving way to student-centered, small-group instruction—similar to the "case study" teaching method common in both law and business schools. In your case, you're likely to be assigned to small groups of students—overseen by a faculty member—in which you will focus on specific clinical problems. The aim here is to instill medical knowledge and skills as well as help you build the communication and collaboration skills you'll need as a resident and, ultimately, as a fully licensed physician.

- Fast-moving technological advances have certainly affected the medical school education program. You'll probably use a computerized patient mannequin (or "whole body simulator") to apply the basic sciences you've mastered to a clinical context and refine your diagnostic skills. These simulators, which are easily customized to replicate a wide range of situations, are currently part of the curriculum in most medical schools.

- Another way medical schools employ new technology is with computer-aided instruction and "virtual" patients. Here, you'll apply newfound knowledge and skills via interactive Web-based (or software) programs that simulate complex cases.

To learn more about the specific teaching methods of the medical school(s) you're interested in, please see the applicable school listing in the *Medical School Admission Requirements* website (*www.aamc.org/msar*).

Choosing a Specialty and Applying for Residency

Required courses. Clerkships. Electives. There is a lot occupying your time and energy as you advance through medical school. You also will be considering the career path you'd like to pursue by exploring various options and researching different possibilities.

At the end of your third year and during your final year, some real decisions must be made. At this stage, you will choose a specialty and begin applying to residency programs (the portion of your education that follows graduation from medical school). How will you make your selection, and how will you get in?

Choosing a Specialty

You should begin exploring specialties in your second year of medical school, and there's much to think about. When choosing your specialty, consider the nature of the work, training and residency requirements, your interests, values and skills, characteristics of physicians in the specialty, issues facing professionals in that particular field, and of course, lifestyle and salary factors.

Types of Educational Technologies

Most medical schools use a combination of the following technologies in their educational programs:

Computer-aided instruction
- Enables visualizing complex processes
- Allows independent exploration
- Offers easy access
- Relatively low cost

Virtual patients
- Covers multiple aspects of a clinical encounter
- Offers easy access
- Readily customized

Human Patient Simulation
- Offers active experience
- Engages emotional and sensory learning
- Fosters critical thought and communication

Source: AAMC Handbook

Match Day Ceremonies

You can view live streaming sessions of Match Day Ceremonies at many medical schools. Be sure to look for links on posted on the AAMC's Pre-Med page on Facebook (*www.facebook.com/aamcpremed*) and Twitter (*@AAMCPreMed*) for more details.

So, where should you begin? First, it's best to seek out the guidance of your advisors, such as the student affairs dean or clinical faculty as you investigate your options, and your school likely will offer various workshops and presentations to help you with your decision. In addition, and as mentioned in the first chapter of this guide, you likely will have access to the Careers in Medicine® (CiM) program sponsored by the AAMC. This largely Web-based program—which is available free of charge to students attending AAMC-member medical schools—contains detailed information and interactive tools to help you work through the specialty choice process.

Included in this program are:

- Specialty descriptions
- Residency and training requirements
- Match data
- Workforce statistics
- Compensation
- Links to more than 1,000 specialty associations, journals, and publications

Registration is required for access to the CiM program. For more information, go to *www.aamc.org/careersinmedicine*.

Getting In

Once you have decided on a specialty or specialties of interest (some students choose more than one as some specialties are extremely competitive and difficult to obtain), you must compete for a position. Much like the application process to medical school, you will complete an application, craft a personal statement, submit letters of evaluation, and be interviewed by residency programs. This process usually is facilitated through an application service such as the AAMC's **Electronic Residency Application Service** (ERAS®, *www.aamc.org/eras*), which transmits all related documentation for you.

After you complete the application, you will find out if you've been accepted by (or "matched" with) a residency program. This pairing is facilitated by the **National Resident Matching Program** (NRMP®, *www.nrmp.org*), which uses an algorithm to match students' preferences for specific residency programs with the preferences of residency program directors. The Match results are released during the third week in March. The third Friday in March—more commonly known as "Match Day"—is met with a great deal of anticipation as 17,000 medical school seniors learn where they will spend the next several years of their training.*

Graduate Medical Education (GME): The Residency Program

Once you have graduated from medical school, you can claim title to that hard-earned M.D. (or D.O. for osteopathic school graduates). Although people now call you "doctor," technically, you're a "doctor in training." The next phase is graduate medical education (GME), or, your residency program.

We won't go into detail about postgraduate work here, as you likely are more interested in getting into medical school now and can focus on your residency program later. In a nutshell, the primary purpose of these programs is to provide medical school graduates

These 17,000 students are the graduates of medical schools that grant the M.D. In addition, 18,000 graduates of osteopathic (those granting the D.O.), Canadian, and international medical schools also compete for residency program assignments through the NRMP. To learn more about ERAS and NRMP, go to www.aamc.org/eras and www.nrmp.org.

U.S. Residents by Specialty

Specialty	# of Residents
Allergy and Immunology	286
Anesthesiology	5,507
Colon and Rectal Surgery	70
Dermatology	1,191
Emergency Medicine	5,458
Family Medicine	9,934
Hospice and Palliative Medicine	164
Internal Medicine	22,710
Medical Genetics	78
Neurological Surgery	1,229
Neurology	2,051
Nuclear Medicine	109
Obstetrics and Gynecology	4,931
Ophthalmology	1,343
Orthopedic Surgery	3,501
Otolaryngology	1,445
Pain Medicine	280
Pathology-Anatomic and Clinical	2,282
Pediatrics	8,332
Physical Medicine and Rehabilitation	1,224
Plastic Surgery	335
Plastic Surgery-Integrated*	438
Preventive Medicine	285
Psychiatry	4,826
Radiation Oncology	663
Radiology-Diagnostic	4,438
Sleep Medicine	136
Surgery-General	7,828
Thoracic Surgery	212
Thoracic Surgery-Integrated*	58
Urology	1,141

Source: AAMC Data Book, 2014, for the 2012–13 academic year

* Integrated programs differ from subspecialty programs in that they include core surgical education.

The most popular subspecialties in internal medicine include:
- Cardiovascular disease (2,514)
- Gastroenterology (1,407)
- Hematology and Oncology (1,531)
- Pulmonary disease and critical care medicine (1,444)
- Nephrology (928)

with the skills and knowledge they need to become competent, independent physicians. Residencies range in length from three to eight years, sometimes more, and program completion is necessary for board certification.

Residency programs are conducted primarily in clinical settings—hospitals, outpatient clinics, community health centers, and physicians' offices, for example—and require residents to participate fully in patient diagnoses and treatment. You will work under the supervision of physician faculty as you develop experience in your chosen specialty, become proficient with both common and uncommon illnesses and conditions, attend conferences, teach less experienced colleagues, and, in general, adjust to the demands of practicing medicine.

Finally, just as medical schools vary, so do residency programs. Depending on the specialty area you choose to pursue, you might complete a preliminary year of broad clinical training before focusing on your specialty. This practice is common in anesthesiology, dermatology, and radiology. In other areas, such as family medicine and pediatrics, you will directly enter the specialty track. (Your medical school advisor and the Careers in Medicine program can provide more information as you approach this stage of your medical education.)

Residency can be a challenging, but rewarding stage of your career. Many physicians look back on their residency years as ones providing invaluable lessons that they carry with them to this day.

Interprofessional Education

When it comes to caring for patients, remember—you're not in this alone.

The delivery of medical care is increasingly a team-based, collaborative effort that includes doctors, nurses, pharmacists, physical therapists, and other health care providers. Caring for a patient effectively and efficiently depends upon practitioners from all disciplines becoming familiar with one another's roles, perspectives, languages, and communication styles.

Because medical educators want to help you develop that knowledge and ability, your medical education is likely to involve some form of "interprofessional education." You will learn to share resources, work as a unit, or participate in other activities that encourage interaction among various categories of health care providers. Through these exercises, you will all become more adept and successful working as a team and, ultimately, be able to deliver high-quality patient care.

Licensure and Certification: Ready to Function Independently

Because all graduates from accredited medical schools must share the same fundamental concepts, before you can be licensed as a physician, you must meet the standards of the **National Board of Medical Examiners®** (NBME®) and the **Federation of State Medical Boards** (FSMB). Together, these two bodies cosponsor the **United States Medical Licensing Examination** (USMLE), a three-step exam given at various stages of the medical education process.

So, along with documenting that you've completed the necessary educational and training programs for your specialty, you also must demonstrate your understanding by earning passing scores on the USMLE exam, which is the final assessment of your ability to assume independent responsibility for delivering medical care and is administered in stages as follows:

- **Step 1:** Usually taken at the end of your second year of medical school, Step 1 tests whether you understand and can apply sciences basic to the practice of medicine. Its focus is on principles and systems of health, disease, and methods of therapy.

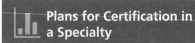

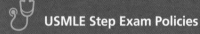
- **Step 2:** Many medical schools require you to take (and pass) Step 2 prior to graduation. It's actually two tests in one—the first evaluates your clinical knowledge (CK) and the second your clinical skills (CS). Basically, Step 2 assesses your ability to provide patient care under supervision.

- **Step 3:** After you've completed the first year of your residency program, you are eligible for Step 3—the concluding test that determines your readiness to apply your medical knowledge and clinical skills without supervision, with an emphasis on patient management in ambulatory settings.

It is the final assessment of your ability to assume independent responsibility for delivering medical care.

After you complete your educational and training programs and achieve passing scores on the USMLE exam, you will be ready to apply for licensure in any of the 50 states, 10 Canadian provinces, three U.S. territories, or the District of Columbia.

But...there is one additional step: certification. While it's not required for medical practice—as is licensure from a state or provincial medical board—certification in a specialty is strongly encouraged. Physicians apply voluntarily for this additional credential, which is granted by the American Board of Medical Specialties (ABMS) and involves a comprehensive exam. (Those who have satisfied all ABMS requirements are certified and are known as "diplomates" of the specialty board.) More than 75 percent of licensed physicians in the United States have been certified by one of the specialty boards, and interest remains high among the current cohort of new doctors. Almost nine in 10 medical school graduates plan to become certified in a medical specialty.

Continuing Medical Education (CME): Lifelong Learning

Finally, as you likely have realized, your medical education will be a lifelong process. As medicine continues to advance and change, you will be provided with the opportunity to learn new skills to stay current with exciting and innovative developments.

The fast pace of change in medicine makes continuing education essential, and most states require participation in accredited continuing medical education (CME) activities. Physicians therefore participate in CME programs throughout their careers, ensuring they stay up-to-date with the rapid advancements in their specialties and maintain their clinical competence. Offered by medical schools, teaching hospitals, and professional organizations, these CME programs are reviewed by the **Accreditation Council for Continuing Medical Education** (ACCME) to ensure that high standards are achieved and upheld.

CME reflects a commitment to lifelong learning that is a hallmark of the medical profession. For those interested in what your CME efforts will entail, go to *www.accme.org*.

Chapter 4:

All About the MCAT® Exam

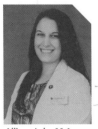

Allison Lyle, M.A.
M.D. Candidate
University of Louisville
School of Medicine
Class of 2017

After my third unsuccessful attempt as a medical school applicant, I was at the point of giving up all hope. With my husband's encouragement, I prepared for my fourth and final application, no matter the outcome.

The feedback I received from several medical schools about my previous applications indicated that I should retake the Medical College Admission Test® (MCAT®) to strengthen my application. Being several years beyond college and science classes, I was apprehensive about taking the exam, but I was hopeful that if I studied and prepared enough, I could earn a higher score and make myself a more competitive candidate.

On the morning of my test date, I was embarrassed to be taking this exam again, which only increased my feelings of inadequacy. However, once I arrived at my exam location I was surprised and comforted to find that several of my fellow examinees were also retaking the exam.

Taking the exam more than once is not recommended for everyone. In my case, thankfully, this exam went well, and I am now a second-year medical student.

MCAT® Essentials: A Must-Read!

To be sure that you get the most complete and up-to-date information about the MCAT® exam, it is crucial that you read **MCAT® Essentials** (available online at *www.aamc.org/mcat*) prior to registration.

The Role of the MCAT Exam

Simply put, the MCAT exam helps admissions officers identify which students are likely to succeed in medical school. That's done by spotting those students who not only have a basic knowledge of the natural, behavioral, and social sciences, which provides the foundation necessary in the early years of medical school, but also those with strong critical analysis and reasoning skills.

One can argue that college grades essentially do the same thing. But because an "A" in one school is not necessarily equivalent to an "A" in another, admissions officers do not have a "standard measure" against which to evaluate students. The MCAT exam fills that void.

It's no surprise, then, that when admissions officers look at MCAT scores in conjunction with grades—as opposed to grades alone—their ability to predict who will be successful in medical school increases substantially.*

See Julian, E. (2005) and Dunleavy, D.M., Kroopnick, M.H., Dowd, K.W., Searcy, C.A,. & Zhao, X (2013). As a result, virtually every medical school in the United States, and many in Canada, requires applicants to submit recent MCAT scores.

How the Exam Is Structured

There are four test sections:

- Biological and Biochemical Foundations of Living Systems

- Chemical and Physical Foundations of Biological Systems

- Psychological, Social, and Biological Foundations of Behavior

- Critical Analysis and Reasoning Skills

Three sections of the test are organized around foundational concepts or "big ideas" in the natural, behavioral, and social sciences. They reflect current research about the most effective ways for students to learn and use science, emphasizing deep knowledge of the most important scientific concepts over knowledge simply of many discrete scientific facts.

Science education leaders say that some of the most important foundational concepts in the sciences ask students to integrate and analyze information from different disciplines. In that vein, questions in these sections will ask you to combine your scientific knowledge from multiple disciplines with your scientific inquiry and reasoning skills. You will be asked to demonstrate four different scientific inquiry and reasoning skills on the exam:

- Knowledge of scientific concepts and principles

- Scientific reasoning and problem solving

- Reasoning about the design and execution of research

- Data-based and statistical reasoning

The fourth section, Critical Analysis and Reasoning Skills, will be similar to many of the verbal reasoning tests you've taken in your academic career. It includes passages and questions that test your ability to comprehend and analyze what you read. This section asks you to read and think about passages from a wide range of disciplines in the social sciences and humanities, including population health, ethics and philosophy, and studies of diverse cultures. Passages are followed by a series of questions that lead you through the process of comprehending, analyzing, and reasoning about the material you have read. This section is unique because it was developed specifically to measure the analytical and reasoning skills you will need to be successful in medical school.

What the Exam Measures

The different sections of the MCAT exam are carefully designed to test the concepts and skills most needed by entering medical students.

The Biological and Biochemical Foundations of Living Systems and the Chemical and Physical Foundations of Biological Systems sections are designed to:

- Test introductory-level biology, organic and inorganic chemistry, and physics concepts

- Test biochemistry concepts at the level taught in many colleges and universities in first-semester biochemistry courses

- Test cellular (Biological and Biochemical Foundations of Living Systems section only) and molecular biology topics at the level taught in many colleges and universities in introductory biology sequences and first-semester biochemistry courses

- Target basic research methods and statistics concepts described by many baccalaureate faculty as important to success in introductory science courses

- Have you demonstrate your scientific inquiry and reasoning, research methods, and statistics skills as applied to the natural sciences

The Psychological, Social, and Biological Foundations of Behavior section is designed to:

- Test your knowledge and use of the concepts in psychology, sociology, and biology that provide a solid foundation for learning about the behavioral and sociocultural determinants of health in medical school

- Target concepts taught at many colleges and universities in first-semester psychology and sociology courses

- Target biology concepts that relate to mental processes and behavior that are taught at many colleges and universities in introductory biology

- Target basic research methods and statistics concepts described by many baccalaureate faculty as important to success in introductory science courses

- Have you demonstrate your scientific inquiry and reasoning, research methods, and statistics skills as applied to the social and behavioral sciences

The Critical Analysis and Reasoning Skills section is designed to:

- Test your comprehension, analysis, and reasoning skills by asking you to critically analyze information provided in reading passages

- Include content from ethics, philosophy, studies of diverse cultures, population health, and a wide range of social sciences and humanities disciplines

- Provide all of the information you need to answer questions in the passages

MCAT Scores

You will receive five results from your MCAT exam: one for each of the four sections and one combined, total score.

Section Scores

Each of the four sections—Biological and Biochemical Foundations of Living Systems; Chemical and Physical Foundations of Biological Systems; Psychological, Social, and Biological Foundations of Behavior; and Critical Analysis and Reasoning Skills—is scored from a low of 118 to a high of 132, with a midpoint of 125. You will receive a score for each of the four sections.

Total Score

Your scores for the four sections are combined to create your total score. The total score ranges from 472 to 528. The midpoint is 500.

For example, if you scored 128 on the Biological and Biochemical Foundations of Living Systems section; 125 on the Chemical and Physical Foundations of Biological Systems section; 129 on the Psychological, Social, and Biological Foundations of Behavior section; and 127 on the Critical Analysis and Reasoning Skills section, your total score would be 509.

Confidence Bands

Like other standardized tests, the MCAT exam is an imperfect measure of what test takers know and can do. Examinees' scores can be affected by factors like fatigue, test anxiety, and less than optimal test-room conditions. Conversely, they can be boosted by recent exposure to some of the tested topics. The use of confidence bands reminds score users to use scores in a way that recognizes the inherent imperfections in the test.

Validity of My MCAT Scores

Each medical school sets its own policy about what it will accept in terms of the age of MCAT scores. To find out specifically how long a school will accept MCAT scores, contact the school(s) you are interested in directly or visit the *Medical School Admission Requirements* website at *www.aamc.org/msar*.

International Students

If you are an international student, you are welcome to take the MCAT exam provided that you meet the eligibility requirements described. If you are in an MBBS (Bachelor of Medicine/ Bachelor of Surgery) degree program or hold the MBBS degree, you may register for the MCAT exam without seeking special permission.

Preparing for the Exam

While there is no one way to prepare for the MCAT exam, making sure you give yourself adequate time to prepare is critical. The amount of time you will need really depends on you. Have you completed all of the coursework that is associated with the content on the exam? Do you feel confident in all content areas? Are there some content topics or skills that you feel require more in-depth study or practice? Are you comfortable with the online testing format?

You may find it useful to break down studying into manageable chunks, realizing that you can't tackle everything at once. This also will help give you a sense of the amount of time you will need so you can prepare at a comfortable pace. The best study plans are those that are tailored to an individual's needs.

Test Dates, Registration, and Fees

In 2015, the MCAT exam will be administered 14 times from April through September. (Specific dates are listed on the *MCAT Exam Schedule* page, posted on the MCAT website at *www.aamc.org/mcat*.) While the AAMC selects exam dates to ensure that scores are available to meet most medical school application deadlines, we recommend that you check the specific scheduling requirements of the school(s) of your choice, provided in the *Medical School Admission Requirements* website (*www.aamc.org/msar*) school profiles. Once you've determined your preferred date, you can find the registration schedule for that particular exam session on the *Registration Deadline Schedule*, also posted online.

After you've read the MCAT Essentials (*www.aamc.org/mcat*), you can register for the exam online through the MCAT website. There is a $300 fee for each exam you take, a payment that covers both the cost of the test itself as well as distribution of your scores. If you register late, make changes to your registration, and/or test at an international site, there are additional charges.

As a general rule, you should plan on taking the MCAT exam 12 to 18 months prior to your expected entry into medical school—but not before you have completed basic coursework and are comfortable with your knowledge of general biology, inorganic and organic chemistry, first-semester biochemistry, general physics, introductory psychology, and introductory sociology. Many medical schools prefer that applicants take the exam in the spring because of the short time between the availability of late summer scores and school application deadlines. (Taking the exam in the spring also allows time for students to retake the test later in the summer, if necessary.) For more guidance, please see your pre-health advisor.

A C/a)∞

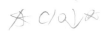

Now ⊗√

Financial Help Available

Cost should not be a barrier to aspiring doctors. The AAMC Fee Assistance Program (FAP) helps qualifying examinees with MCAT registration fees, test preparation products, and other AAMC complimentary products and services. Learn if you might qualify for FAP at *https://www.aamc.org/students/applying/fap/*.

Register as early as you can

Carefully selecting your preferred testing dates and locations and then registering *as early as possible* will provide the best opportunity to select your top choice for an MCAT exam date and site. The Gold Zone registration period provides the greatest flexibility and lowest fees. As an examinee, you will see decreasing test site and test date availability and increased fees in the Silver and Bronze Zone registration periods. Visit *www.aamc.org/students/applying/mcat/reserving* for details.

What Does My Advisor Suggest?

As you deliberate whether to retake the MCAT exam—or any number of other questions concerning medical school admissions—make sure you ask your pre-health advisor for guidance. He or she will have recommendations to help make your decision easier.

Don't have an advisor? The National Association of Advisors for the Health Professions (NAAHP) has volunteer advisors. More information is available at *www.naahp.org*.

Testing with Accommodations

The AAMC is committed to providing all individuals with an opportunity to demonstrate their proficiency on the MCAT exam, and that includes ensuring access to persons with disabilities in accordance with relevant law.

If you have a disability or medical condition that you believe requires an adjustment to the standard testing conditions, we encourage you to apply for accommodated testing. If you plan to test with accommodations, be sure to allow enough time between submitting your accommodation application and your registered test date in order to get an answer regarding your accommodation application prior to your registered test date.

Information about the process by which accommodations are requested (and the documentation that should accompany the request) is available at *www.aamc.org/mcat/accommodations*.

Retaking the Exam

If you are not happy with your performance on the MCAT exam, you have the option to take it again. But it's a tough decision.

There are times when a retake is well worth considering. Perhaps you discovered that your coursework or study didn't cover the topics as thoroughly as you needed. Or there's a large discrepancy between your grade in a subject and your score on a particular section. Or maybe you simply didn't feel well the day of the exam. In all these cases, your pre-health advisor may be of great help, and we recommend you discuss the issue with him or her.

Score Reporting

Your scores will be available in the MCAT Score Reporting System (SRS) accessible through the AAMC website at *www.aamc.org/mcat*. You have several options for sending your MCAT scores to medical schools.

- **Send your scores to AMCAS service:**
  As mentioned, the AMCAS® service is the American Medical College Application Service®, in which most U.S. medical schools take part, and the process by which you will manage sending your application to participating institutions. Through this system, MCAT scores are submitted to each school on your application list. You can view a list of participating schools at *www.aamc.org/amcas*.

- **Send your scores to non-AMCAS schools:**
  Use this option, detailed in the MCAT Score Reporting System, to send your MCAT scores to non-AMCAS schools and programs.

What's AMCAS?

AMCAS is a nonprofit, centralized application processing service in which most U.S. medical schools take part, and the process by which you will manage your application (to participating institutions). Through this system, scores are submitted to each school you've designated. For more information, see Chapter 6, which discusses the AMCAS application process in detail.

The MCAT exam is administered and scored by the MCAT Program Office at the direction of the AAMC. Information about the exam's content, organization, scoring system, accommodations process, and more, is available at www.aamc.org/mcat.

Chapter 5:

Choosing the Schools That Are Right for You

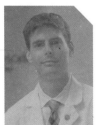

Matthew Joy, M.D.
Virginia Tech Carilion
School of Medicine,
Class of 2014
Resident, General
Surgery, Virginia Tech
Carilion School of
Medicine

With so many schools to choose from, applicants should carefully consider what kind of medical education experience they are seeking. When I was researching medical schools, geographic location was an obvious consideration, but it also was important to look at things like class size, grading systems (pass-fail versus traditional), teaching styles (lecture hall versus small groups), research requirements, as well as locations for third- and fourth-year clinical rotations.

Once I was in medical school, I realized the importance of figuring out which school offers a learning environment that is most in line with your style of learning and educational needs. For example, some applicants may desire smaller class sizes and small-group learning. Some students prefer programs with more structure and direct guidance, whereas others may thrive in larger group settings that offer more freedom to direct the course of their own education.

Once you determine your preferences, make a list that includes information about your considerations for each school you want to apply to so you can compare schools based on the criteria that matter most to you and your educational needs. This is a great time to use the Medical School Admission Requirements website (www.aamc. org/msar), where you can sort and compare school profiles based on class size, requirements, and a myriad of other factors. Finally, whenever you have the opportunity to visit a school during the application process, be sure to ask about the things on your list to get the current student, faculty, and administration perspective.

In this chapter, you will learn about some important factors to consider when choosing the school that's right for you.

The Overall Mission of the School

If you've seen one medical school…you've seen one medical school. And many of the differences among schools are obvious. Some schools are located in the East; some in the West. Some are private; others, public. Some have a large entering class; others, small. And, as explained in Chapter 3, medical schools vary in the content of their courses, in the way they teach, and even in the way they grade and evaluate students.

These are all factors you'll want to consider as you narrow your selection, and we touch upon them in the following pages. But the differences go even deeper and at a very core level: medical schools have diverse missions and priorities. Because of these distinctions, what is significant to one school may be of only moderate importance to another, and these goals naturally carry into the selection process.

Deciding where to apply requires that you become aware of the differences among schools, which is crucial, but it's also important to analyze yourself—your skills, experiences, career

Students Weigh a Host of Selection Factors

There's much to take into account when choosing schools. Among the factors medical students consider in making their ultimate selection as to which school to attend are:

- Advice of medical school graduates
- Advice of family physician
- Research reputation and opportunities
- Community-based experience and opportunities
- Geographic location
- School's teaching methods
- Program of elective courses
- Faculty mentorship
- Ability of school to place students in particular residency programs

Source: AAMC's 2014 Matriculating Student Questionnaire (MSQ)

About the Medical School Interview

Remember that the medical school interview is a two-way evaluation. You are judging whether the school is the best "fit" for you, while the admissions committee members are judging whether you are a good fit for the school. Look upon your interview, then, as an opportunity to answer some remaining questions you may have about the school. Read about medical school interviews in Chapter 7.

goals, and so forth—to identify the most appropriate matches. Take, for instance, an institution that places a strong emphasis on primary care. Is that the career path you intend to follow? If so, and especially if you can demonstrate your interest through extensive experience related to that area, you become a more attractive candidate on that basis alone.

That's one example. Other schools may be actively seeking students from specific geographic or rural areas. Others may be looking for students with a high potential for a research career. Still others may want to increase the number of doctors who plan to practice in their state (this last goal is often found among public institutions). The differing missions among schools will be reflected in their admissions policies and standards.

If you need help with this self-analysis, think back to the various experiences you've had over the years. The ones you found especially rewarding or inspirational are likely to correlate to a specific area of interest and, by extension, a career goal.

Did you volunteer for two summers at a clinic in a **rural, underserved area**? Perhaps that's the direction you'd like to take your career. If so, you'll want to seek out medical schools that place a high priority in that area.

Were the part-time jobs you had while doing research particularly gratifying? If you'd like to pursue a **research career**, look for schools that have a strong reputation in that area or are known for graduating a large percentage of medical students pursuing research careers.

There are also other ways that speak to your interests and career goals. Did you spend your junior year tutoring freshmen and sophomores in entry-level biology or chemistry? Perhaps you'd like to join a **medical school faculty** and educate the next generation of physicians. If so, look for a medical school with a relatively large percentage of their graduates in teaching positions.

Once again, keep in mind that applying to medical school is a two-way street. While you're looking for a match, so are the schools. Your experiences will provide good insights for the admissions officers and help them determine if your interests and their missions are congruent. If you don't know which medical career path you want to pursue yet, that's okay. Aim to get as many rich and diverse experiences as possible so you will be a well-rounded applicant.

Kicking Off Your Research

There are several ways you can research schools to identify the ones that best match your own strengths, interests, and goals.

The *Medical School Admission Requirements* website: Start with the medical school profiles on this site (*www.aamc.org/msar*). Here, each institution includes a clear mission statement and a description of its selection factors.

School websites and literature: You'll also want to review information provided by schools themselves. Although the specific content varies by school, each includes detailed material for prospective students.

Advisors: Your pre-health advisor or career counselor will be able to recommend specific schools likely to be a good "fit." These advisors have a lot of insight about the application process, so don't overlook this resource. Also, make sure you attend health career fairs to speak with admissions staff from medical schools and participate in premed or pre-health student organizations.

factors - I

The Educational Program

It's easy to get caught up in a specific region or location, but as you weigh your decision, you'll also want to consider the differences among the educational programs themselves.

There's likely going to be a strong relationship between a school's mission and its **curriculum**. You'll be able to gauge whether an institution's objectives align with your interests by analyzing course requirements and electives programs. A medical school with a mission to graduate more primary care doctors may, for example, have a track that provides additional training in that area. A school that emphasizes research may require their students to write a thesis or devote an extended period of time to scholarly pursuits.

Yes!
No?
PITT - BOTH!

As you do your research, also consider what **teaching methods** you find most effective. Do you tend to do well with self-directed or participatory learning exercises, or do you prefer a learning environment with the more traditional, lecture-based style? While most medical schools use an educational model that combines a variety of methods, every program adapts their own design. Are you looking for classes that promote small-group discussions and problem-based learning exercises? Or are you more comfortable with a traditional teaching approach? Eventually, these are great topics to discuss with current students, but a good starting point for your exploration is a school's website, as well as the AAMC's curriculum directory (*https://www.aamc.org/initiatives/cir/*).

There are key differences among **grading systems**. Some institutions use a pass/fail system or an honors/pass/fail system, while others use letter grades. Some students have definite preferences, and if you're one of them, you may wish to consider a school's grading system as you narrow your selection.

There are many other factors you might want to think about. How will you be evaluated? At what point must students pass the first two steps of the United States Medical Licensing Examination (USMLE) before advancing in their education? What level of academic support is available? Is there a mentor system, for instance? What about support services or organizations for cultural and other minorities—are they available? Questions such as these will undoubtedly enter into your final decision as you deliberate among offers.

How Do GPA and MCAT Scores Factor In?

Don't choose schools based solely on where you think your grades and MCAT scores will be accepted. While there's no question that your educational record is important and that admissions officers seek candidates who are likely to succeed academically in their programs, it's important to realize that **academics alone do not predict who will become an effective physician, and admissions officers know that all too well.**

The fact that there are many instances in which a "high scoring" applicant is not accepted to a medical school—and in which an applicant with lower-than-average grades and scores is—tells you that admissions officers must be looking at other factors.

Admissions officers are taking a more "holistic" approach to evaluating applicants. Through this practice, admissions officers assess candidates more broadly, looking not only at their "metrics" (GPA and MCAT scores) but also at their experiences and personal attributes.

You can read about the holistic approach to admissions in Chapter 7: "*The Admissions Decision.*"

school's decision

Attending Medical School in Your "Home" State

[handwritten margin note: Only → public state schools]

State residents enrolled in state-supported medical schools pay lower tuition than nonresidents. In addition, in-state residents often are given preference for admission (compared to out-of-state residents) for at least some of their spaces because the school receives state government support. With this in mind, you may want to give strong consideration to the public institutions in your state as you decide where to apply.

Nationally, 61 percent of 2014 matriculants attended schools in their home state.

Public or Private?

You also may be deliberating between public and private institutions. Typically, the most cost-effective option is to consider a public medical school in your state of residence. (If you're from out of state, the cost differential between a public and private school virtually disappears. See chart in Chapter 11.) But don't automatically assume, even if you are interested in a state school near your home, that the private route will be more expensive under all circumstances. Some private institutions have large endowments that allow them to provide significant scholarship aid to qualifying students. These scholarships lower the "effective" tuition rate and permit those students to graduate with less educational debt than they would have generated if they had attended a public medical school in their home state.

But cost is only one consideration. Another element to be aware of when investigating the differences between private and public institutions is the school's mission—and how it might relate to your own aspirations and interests. Although all medical schools—public or private—have different missions, certain public institutions may have specific goals related to their state, such as increasing the supply of physicians. (If the school is in your home state and you'd like to live and work there after graduation, that will be a factor from both your perspective and the school's.) Other public institutions were founded by state legislators with an emphasis on the needs of a particular patient population—such as elder, rural, or underserved groups—which should enter into your evaluation if that objective corresponds to your own career intentions.

Additional Factors to Consider

There are many other factors that may be important to you as you search for a good "match." Some of these include:

- *Location*

    Perhaps you simply prefer a specific geographic region. Do you want to be close to family and friends? Do you prefer a warmer (or cooler) climate? Are you a fan of the East coast...or the South...or the West? What about a bustling city environment versus a rural one? These factors play to your comfort level, and are all valid considerations. Beyond that, though, location can also relate to your career goals, as well as to a school's mission. If you hope to specialize in geriatrics, for example, a medical school located in an area with a higher-than-average proportion of older adults may be able to provide you with the experience you seek.

    That's looking at it from your perspective. Consider, for a moment, the school's perspective. In some cases, a school may be seeking students from particular geographic regions in order to bolster its diversity, and you'll want to consider the impact—if any—that your own state residence might have on your application to medical schools in other areas.

• *Size and Demographics*

The size and demographics of the medical school—both in terms of its student body as well as its faculty—may be a consideration for you, as well. The school entries in the *Medical School Admission Requirements* website (*www.aamc.org/msar*) include data on the prior year's entering class, including the number of students by gender as well as by self-reported identification.

• *Costs*

Medical education is expensive and the expenses associated with particular institutions will no doubt be a factor in your decision. You won't know what your actual costs will be (or the degree of assistance you will receive) until a school sends you a financial aid package in conjunction with its offer. Still, in looking through the school entries in the *Medical School Admission Requirements* website, you can get a general idea as to the relative expenses of each institution, and you can take those numbers into consideration as you narrow your selection.

Special Regional Opportunities

Finally, you should be aware that some states without a public medical school participate in special interstate and regional agreements which provide their residents with access to a medical education. Currently, there are five interstate agreements, listed below:

• The Delaware Institute of Medical Information and Research
  http://dhss.delaware.gov/dhss/dhcc/dimer.html
  1-302-577-3240
  1-800-292-7935

• The Finance Authority of Maine's Access to Medical Education Program
  www.famemaine.com/files/Pages/education/students_and_families/Medical_Education.aspx
  1-800-228-3734

• University of Utah School of Medicine Idaho Contract
  http://medicine.utah.edu/admissions/begin/residency.php
  1-208-282-2475,
  residency@sa.utah.edu

• The Western Interstate Commission for Higher Education
  www.wiche.edu/psep/medi
  1-303-541-0200

• The WWAMI (Washington, Wyoming, Alaska, Montana, and Idaho) Program
  http://uwmedicine.washington.edu/Education/WWAMI/Pages/Medical-School.aspx

You can learn more about each of these regional opportunities by visiting their websites or calling their program offices.

Chapter 6

Applying to Medical School

include all in this chapter overview (handwritten)

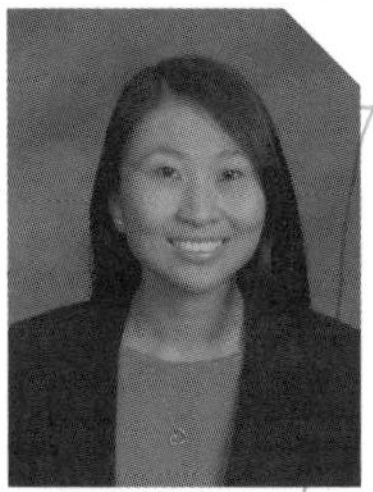

Amanda Xi
Oakland University
William Beaumont
(OUWB) School of
Medicine
Class of 2015

As you embark on your journey to medical school, there may be moments when you feel overwhelmed, anxious, or frustrated. In those moments, take a couple deep breaths and remind yourself that it's all worth it.

One of those moments may come when it's time to complete your medical school applications. In preparation for the application season, I met with my pre-health advisor for tips on how to stay organized and learn about the resources available. I learned that AMCAS® (the American Medical College Application Service®) is used by almost every medical school in the country. To keep myself from feeling overwhelmed before starting my AMCAS application, I read through the instruction manual to ensure that I was familiar with the system. From there, I requested transcripts, asked for letters of evaluation, and started a spreadsheet to keep track of schools, secondary applications, and notes from my interviews and communication with each school.

My recommendations for applicants are:

1. *Work with your letter writers to set deadlines that allow them enough time to write high-quality letters, but also ensure that you comfortably meet your deadlines.*

2. *Prior to submitting **anything**—requests for letters, your personal statement, your AMCAS application—save a draft and reread it at a later time.*

3. *Take a deep breath and slowly exhale. When you feel overwhelmed in the moment, consider how gratifying your career in medicine will be. Although the application process is arduous, with adequate preparation and organization, it will fly by in a blur!*

Responsibilities of the Medical School Applicant

As an applicant, you have certain responsibilities when it comes to applying to medical school. These are reviewed at length at the end of this chapter, but some of the most critical are:

- Meeting all deadlines
- Completing the AMCAS application accurately
- Knowing the admission requirements at each school
- Promptly updating your AMCAS application with any change in contact information
- Responding promptly to interview invitations

If you have previously registered for the MCAT® exam, the Fee Assistance Program, or other AAMC services, you already created an AAMC username and password and received an AAMC ID. **Use this same access information to enter the AMCAS application site**. If you do not already have an AAMC ID number, you will need to register online to create a username and password before you begin your application. Visit *www.aamc.org/amcas* when you're ready to begin the application process.

- Filing for financial aid as soon as possible

- Withdrawing from the schools you will not attend

For details, see "AAMC's Application and Acceptance Protocols – Applicants" later in this chapter.

American Medical College Application Service® (AMCAS®)

You may have heard about the American Medical College Application Service (AMCAS) from your pre-health advisor, career counselor, or even your classmates. AMCAS is a centralized medical school application processing service offered by the AAMC and utilized by almost every medical school in the country. (For information about schools that do not participate in AMCAS, see the non-AMCAS schools box later in this chapter.) This service does not screen applicants; rather, it provides admissions officers with the information and tools they need to select the applicants who are the best fit for their institution.

AMCAS provides many benefits to applicants. The most obvious one is that it allows you to apply to as many medical schools as you want with a single application (although many schools require a secondary application, a topic discussed later in this chapter). It also provides applicants with a single point of transmission for official transcripts, letters of evaluation, and other supporting documentation.

Even if you're not yet ready to begin the application process, you can familiarize yourself with the process at *www.aamc.org/amcas*. There, you'll find information on the key steps involved in starting an application, an application overview, tips useful in completing the application, answers to frequently asked questions, and a comprehensive instruction manual.

AMCAS Application Sections

The AMCAS application is organized into nine sections. That might sound like a lot, but remember, you don't have to complete it all at once. You can save your work and return to your application as many times as you want until you finish and are ready to submit it. Here's an overview of what to expect:

1. **Identifying Information.** This section asks you to enter your name, birth information, and sex.

2. **Schools Attended.** Here, you will enter high school and college information. Once this section (and the identifying information section) is completed, you will be able to create a Transcript Request Form, which will help you request official transcripts from your registrar.

3. **Biographic Information.** You will use this section to enter your contact information, citizenship status, legal residence, ethnicity, language(s) spoken, and other biographic information.

4. **Course Work.** You will enter grades and credits for every course that you have enrolled in at any U.S., U.S. territorial, or Canadian postsecondary institution. (You are required to provide information for all the college-level courses you've taken, even if taken during high school.)

5. **Work/Activities.** Here, you will enter any work and extracurricular activities, awards, honors, or publications that you would like to bring to the attention of the medical school(s). You may list up to 15 experiences.

Letters of Evaluation

Review the AAMC's Letters of Evaluation Guidelines. This is a useful tool to provide to your letter writers: *https://www.aamc.org/ initiatives/admissionsinitiative/letters/*

6. **Letters of Evaluation.** In this section, you will provide information about people writing letters of evaluation on your behalf. (This step is covered in more detail later in the chapter.)

7. **Medical Schools.** In this section, you will designate the medical schools to which you want to submit an application. In addition, you can designate which letters of evaluation you wish to send to specific schools.

8. **Personal Statement.** Here, you will compose an essay about why you want to go to medical school. (This is discussed more thoroughly later in this chapter.)

9. **Standardized Tests.** And finally…your MCAT® scores. In this section, you will review your MCAT scores and enter any additional test information such as GRE scores. Please note that MCAT scores earned in 2003 or later will automatically be released to AMCAS, and no further action will be required on your part.

Of course, this is just a simplified overview of the AMCAS application. Read the AMCAS Instruction Manual and explore the various resources for a more thorough understanding of the application on the AMCAS website at *www.aamc.org/amcas*.

Transcript Requests via AMCAS

In addition to completing your AMCAS application, you must request that official transcripts from all postsecondary institutions at which you've registered be sent to AMCAS. AMCAS provides a Transcript Request Form to facilitate this process with your registrar(s). If you have taken courses at a junior college, community college, trade school, or other professional school—regardless of whether credit was earned—within the United States, Canada, or U.S. territories, you must provide an official transcript from that institution. (This requirement also applies to any college courses you took in high school.) For most applicants, all official transcripts must be received no later than two weeks after the deadline date for application materials. Please refer to the AMCAS Instruction Manual and the AMCAS website for detailed information about official transcript requirements.

Limited Changes After Submission

It's important to check your work carefully before you hit "submit" because you're limited in what changes you can make after submission. Although you can make changes to your contact information (such as addresses) and add additional schools or letters of evaluation, your application will be submitted to schools exactly as it was completed.

Application Processing and Verification

Once AMCAS has received your submitted application and all required official transcripts from each postsecondary school where you were registered, AMCAS verification process begins. AMCAS verifies the accuracy of your academic record by comparing the information you entered on your application to that on your official transcripts. During the verification process, AMCAS converts transcript grades to AMCAS grades based on conversion information provided by colleges and universities and calculates an AMCAS GPA. The AMCAS GPA provides medical schools with a standard way to compare each applicant's academic record. AMCAS GPAs may differ from the GPA shown on your records at the institutions you attended. Once verification is complete, AMCAS makes your application and MCAT scores available to all the medical schools you designated. (MCAT scores from 2003 and later are automatically included.)

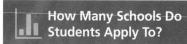

How Many Schools Do Students Apply To?

For the 2015 AMCAS application cycle, students applied to an average of 15.7 schools.

Source: AMCAS® Data

Non-AMCAS Schools

The U.S. medical schools that are not participating in AMCAS for the 2016 entering class are:

- Texas A&M University System Health Science Center College of Medicine*^
- Texas Tech University Health Sciences Center School of Medicine*^
- Texas Tech University Health Sciences Center, El Paso, Paul. L. Foster School of Medicine*
- University of Texas Southwestern Medical Center at Dallas Southwestern Medical School*^
- University of Texas Medical School at Galveston*^
- University of Texas School of Medicine at Houston*^
- University of Texas School of Medicine at San Antonio*^

If you are interested in schools that do not participate in AMCAS, please contact them directly for application instructions.

You should also contact schools directly for application information if you wish to pursue a joint program, such as a B.A.-M.D. or M.D.-Ph.D.

The seven public medical schools in Texas listed here participate in the Texas Medical and Dental School Application Service for those pursuing the M.D. degree. You can learn more about this application service at www.utsystem.edu/tmdsas.

^These schools participate in AMCAS® for those pursuing M.D.-Ph.D. degrees.

The Application and Admissions Cycle

The AMCAS application usually opens to applicants in early May of each year and opens for submission in early June. Participating schools receive verified application data from AMCAS in late June.

The deadlines for receipt of primary applications to medical schools that participate in AMCAS are from mid-October to mid-December. (Information on Secondary Applications is discussed further in this chapter.) However, there is no single application timetable as each school establishes its own deadlines for receipt of required materials. You can find specific dates in medical schools' bulletins and websites and in the school listings on the *Medical School Admission Requirements* website (*www.aamc.org/msar*).

Medical schools vary in the timing of their admissions decisions. Most schools use a system of "rolling admissions," selecting students for interviews and making admissions decisions as applications are received, rather than waiting until after a specific deadline date to begin their evaluation process. All medical schools must wait until mid-October before they can start offering acceptance letters. (You can find out if a medical school uses a rolling admissions system by checking its website.)

As far as interviews go, many admissions committees begin meeting with candidates in the late summer and continuing through spring. However, the majority of interviews are held during the winter months. (This part of the admissions cycle is discussed in Chapter 7.) By March 30, medical schools will have issued enough acceptances at least equal to the size of their first-year entering class.

Personal Statements and Letters of Evaluation

As you will learn in Chapter 7, *The Admissions Decision*, admissions officers want to know more about you than just where you went to college, the courses you've taken, the grades you've earned, and how you scored on the MCAT exam. They want to know you on a more personal level. That's why an essay and letters of evaluation are integral components of your medical school application.

Your Personal Statement

Every applicant is required to submit a Personal Comments essay of up to 5,300 characters (or approximately one page) in length. This is your opportunity to distinguish yourself from other applicants and provide admissions officers with insights about why you're interested in medicine—and why you would be a dedicated and effective physician.

Most admissions committees place significant weight on this section, so take the time to craft an organized, well-written, and compelling statement. Here are some questions you may want to consider while crafting your essay:

- Why do you want a career in medicine?
- What motivates you to learn more about medicine?
- What should medical schools know about you that isn't described in other sections of the application?

In addition, you may wish to include information such as:

- What special hardships, challenges, or obstacles have influenced your educational pursuits?
- Are you able to explain significant fluctuations in your academic record not explained elsewhere in your application?

Early Decision Programs

One of your first decisions will be whether to apply to a medical school through the Early Decision Program (EDP) or the regular application process. Although criteria for accepting EDP applicants vary among schools, the program frequently requires that applicants show extraordinary credentials. A small percentage of applicants apply through the EDP, and only about half of medical schools even offer it. You can learn more about program requirements at *www.aamc.org/students/applying/requirements/edp* and look at each school's EDP policy in the *Medical School Admission Requirements* website.

For M.D.-Ph.D. Applicants

Applicants to M.D.-Ph.D. programs will be required to write two additional essays: a relatively brief one focusing on your reasons for pursuing the combined degree, and a lengthier one (about three pages) describing your research activities. You can read more about these additional essays in the AMCAS Instruction Manual or get further guidance from your pre-health advisor or career counselor.

How to Choose Your Letter Writer

You should seek someone who knows you well and whose opinion is likely to be highly valued. (For example, admissions committees are not likely to place as much value on the input of your teaching assistant, but they will weigh heavily the thoughts of the biology department chair who taught your honors biology class.) These letters can be very valuable, so you should be thoughtful in selecting who you ask to write on your behalf.

It's a good idea to use specific examples in your essay. Instead of writing *"Challenges in my childhood led me to consider medicine at an early age,"* write, *"The summer I turned eight, my 11-year-old sister was diagnosed with Neuroblastoma, and I witnessed firsthand the compassion and understanding with which the doctor dealt with my parents. It was during those first few difficult months that I decided I wanted to be a physician."*

Additionally, ensure that your essay is interesting, follows a logical and orderly flow, and relates to your reasons for choosing medicine and/or why you believe you will be successful in medical school and as a physician. Beyond that, be sure to use correct grammar and avoid typographical errors or misspellings.

Letters of Evaluation

The Letters of Evaluation section requires you to provide information about the people writing your letters of evaluation. While you can add up to 10 letter entries, that does not mean medical schools wish to receive 10 letters for each applicant. Most schools request only two or three letters. (You can find the minimum and maximum letters accepted by each school in the *Medical School Admission Requirements* website.) AMCAS allows additional letters so that you have the option to designate specific letters for specific schools.

Medical schools have various requirements regarding letters of evaluation, but they all require them in one form or another. If your college has a pre-health advisor, medical schools probably will require a letter from him or her (or from the pre-health committee, if your school has one), as well as a letter from at least one faculty member. In instances where there is no pre-health advisor, many medical schools may ask for additional letters from faculty and often specify that at least one comes from a science professor.

Some medical schools do not specify who writes your letters and welcome additional letters beyond those that are required. However, be aware of any limits on the number they will accept. In all cases, you should review medical schools' websites or the *Medical School Admission Requirements* website (*www.aamc.org/msar*) for information on specific letter requirements.

Medical schools want letters from those who are in a position to judge your ability to be successful in medical school, which includes not only your academic capabilities and accomplishments, but also your personal characteristics and skills.

Secondary Applications

Your primary application is your AMCAS application and provides admissions officers with much of the information they need. However, most medical schools also require a school-specific, or "secondary" application because it allows them to assess students' reasons for applying to that particular school. (Medical schools will notify you if they would like you to fill out a secondary application, although you also can find out by looking at their profile in the *Medical School Admission Requirements* website.) Secondary applications may call for additional letters of evaluation, supplemental writing samples, and/or updated transcripts. Go to the websites of the medical schools you are interested to learn more.

Application Fees

Medical school application fees fall into four general categories:

AMCAS Application
For the 2015 application cycle, the AMCAS application fee plus designation to one school was $160, and $36 for each additional school. Check the AMCAS website for the latest

application fee information. (Remember, some schools do not use AMCAS and you may incur a different fee in those instances.)

Secondary Application
In 2014, fees for secondary applications ranged from $0 to $150.

College Service Fees
Your college registrar may charge a small fee to send your transcript to AMCAS. Occasionally, you will incur a fee to send your letters of evaluation to AMCAS.

MCAT Exam Fees
Although technically not an application fee, the costs associated with the MCAT exam are a necessary component of the overall process. Registration for the MCAT exam is $275 and covers the cost of the exam as well as distribution of your scores. In addition, you may incur fees for late registration, changes to your registration, or testing at international test sites. You can read more about the MCAT exam in Chapter 4 and the MCAT website (*www.aamc.org/mcat*).

For more information on application fees, go to *www.aamc.org/first/factsheets*.

Criminal Background Check

The AAMC facilitates a national background check on all accepted applicants to participating medical schools via Certiphi Screening, Inc. (a Vertical Screen® Company). This service provides required background checks to medical schools and prevents you from paying additional fees to each medical school to run these checks independently. For more information, go to *www.aamc.org/amcascbc*.

Be aware that participating medical schools also may require applicants to undergo a separate national background check process, if it's required by their own institutional regulations or by applicable state law.

Fee Assistance Program

The AAMC believes that the cost of applying to medical school should not be a financial barrier to those interested in becoming physicians.

The AAMC Fee Assistance Program assists MCAT examinees and AMCAS applicants who, without financial assistance, would be unable to take the MCAT exam, apply to medical schools that use the AMCAS application, or gain access to the Pivio® System. Visit the Fee Assistance Program website for details about the program eligibility requirements and to access the application.

Fee Assistance Program Award Benefits

Applicants who are approved for fee assistance in 2015 will receive the following:

MCAT Benefits
- Reduced registration fees for up to four MCAT exam dates until December 31, 2016

- Reduced rescheduling fees for MCAT exam dates until December 31, 2016

- A suite of MCAT prep products and resources. You will receive more details about these benefits if you are awarded fee assistance.

- Up to $500 toward an updated psycho-educational or medical evaluation if it is required to support your MCAT accommodations application.

Regardless of how many times you are awarded fee assistance, you will only receive MCAT prep product benefits once.

Medical School Admission Requirements Benefits
- Complimentary access to the *Medical School Admission Requirements* website until December, 31, 2016 ($50 value)

AMCAS Benefits
- Waiver for all AMCAS fees for one application submission with up to 15 medical schools designations ($664 value)

Additional fees will be charged for each medical school designation beyond the initial set of 15.

Pivio Benefits
- Reduced subscription fee to Pivio for up to two years—$25.00 for a one-year subscription from the date of activation ($75 value)

The Pivio system is an electronic portfolio service created by the AAMC and the National Board of Medical Examiners (NBME®) that allows you to organize, archive, and transfer important information throughout your medical career.

Special Note About Deferred Entry

In recent years, most medical schools have developed delayed matriculation policies to allow accepted applicants to defer entry without giving up their spot. Deferrals are granted only after acceptance. These programs usually require that you submit a written request, and some schools also ask for a report at the end of the deferral period. Matriculation delays are usually granted for one year, although some schools occasionally may defer for longer periods of time. Some institutions may require delayed matriculants to sign an agreement to not apply to other medical schools in the interim, while others permit applications to other schools. Interested applicants should seek specific information from schools where they applied. You can find out more about each school's policy by viewing their profile in the *Medical School Admission Requirements* website.

Application and Acceptance Protocols—Applicants

The AAMC recommends the following to help ensure that all M.D. and M.D.-Ph.D. applicants receive timely notification about the outcome of their application and protect schools and programs from having unfilled positions in their entering classes. These protocols often are referred to as "traffic rules" by admissions officers and pre-health advisors. Prospective applicants, their advisors, and admissions staff at medical schools and programs should all be aware of these application and acceptance protocols for applicants.

The AAMC recommends that as an applicant to a M.D. or M.D.-Ph.D. program, you:

1. Understand and comply with these applicant responsibilities as well as with the application, acceptance, and admissions procedures at each school or program to which you apply.

2. Provide accurate and truthful information in all aspects of your application, interview(s), acceptance, and admissions processes for each school or program to which you apply.

3. Submit all application documents (e.g., primary and secondary application forms, transcript(s), letters of evaluation/recommendation, fees, etc.) on or before the school or program's published deadline date.

4. Notify all relevant medical school application services of any change, permanent or temporary, to your contact information (e.g., mailing address, telephone number, and email address).

5. If you will be unavailable for an extended period of time (e.g., during foreign travel, vacation, or holidays) during the application/admission process:

   a. Provide instructions regarding your application and the authority to respond to any offers of acceptance to a parent or other responsible individual in your absence.

   b. Inform all schools or programs at which your application remains under consideration of this person's name and contact information.

6. Respond promptly to a school's or program's invitation for an interview. If you cannot appear for a scheduled interview, notify the school or program **immediately** that you need to cancel via the school or program's preferred method.

7. Begin the steps necessary to determine your eligibility for financial aid. This may include filing need-analysis forms early and having your parents (when required) file the appropriate income tax forms.

8. In fairness to other applicants, if you have decided before April 30 not to attend a medical school or program that has offered you an acceptance, promptly withdraw your application from that school(s) or program(s) by written correspondence or the method preferred.

9. If you receive an offer of acceptance from more than one school or program, choose the school that you will enroll in by April 30. Then, **promptly** withdraw your application, by written correspondence, from all other schools or programs that have offered you an acceptance.

10. Withdraw your application from consideration at all other schools or programs as soon as you enroll, or start an orientation program prior to enrollment, at a U.S. or Canadian school or program.

*If any date falls on a weekend/holiday, the recommendation(s) will apply to the following business day.

Approved by the AAMC Council of Deans Administrative Board, September 2014

Chapter 7

The Admissions Decision

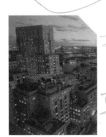

Lori Nicolaysen
Assistant Dean of
Admissions
Weill Cornell Medical
College

Admissions committees agree that while expectations vary from school to school, most are looking for two things: students who can handle challenging academic work, and those who are genuinely good human beings who demonstrate good judgment, compassion, and selflessness—qualities every physician should embody. In my experience, admissions committees also are looking for students who have demonstrated exceptional personal initiative in the form of leadership, creativity, research, community service, motivation, or other life experiences. It sounds simple, but by demonstrating that you can handle rigorous coursework and also exhibit the positive personal attributes needed to work with people conveys to admissions committees that you are the kind of person who should be a doctor.

So how do you do that? Exceling in upper-level courses and doing well on the MCAT® exam shows that you can handle medical school coursework, while demonstrating good judgment, compassion, leadership, and selflessness through your extracurricular involvement, letters of evaluation, and personal statement, which show that you're likely to have the personal qualities of a good physician.

It is important to have a pre-health advisor or other valued colleague read over your application because no matter how closely you think you've checked it, a fresh pair of eyes may find something you missed. Before submitting your application, ask some trusted mentors, friends, or family members to give you feedback about your experiences and essays. You might ask them questions such as, "How would you describe me based on what you read? Did my essay hold your attention? Was anything confusing? Did you notice any typos?"

It is incredibly challenging for committees to choose among applicants because there are so many admirable candidates. Ultimately, the committee screeners attempt to identify the applicants most likely to succeed academically, build a dynamic and diverse learning environment at the medical school, care for patients diligently, and become leaders in medicine.

The Holistic Review of Medical School Applicants

What does holistic mean, and how does it affect the admissions review process?

Holistic review is a flexible, individualized way of assessing an applicant. The review considers a balance of an applicant's experiences, attributes, and academic metrics (E-A-M) and, when taken together, how the individual may contribute value as a medical student and future physician. When admissions committees select individual applicants, they intentionally try to create a broadly diverse class to help fulfill their school's mission.

Each medical school's admissions office evaluates applicants based upon the mission, goals, and diversity interests of their institution. They must decide which applicants will best

Depth…not Breadth!

As mentioned in Chapter 2, a series of short-term involvements (volunteering a day here, spending an afternoon there, and so forth) does not really convey a true interest in the area, and this underlying motivation is transparent to admissions officers. They are looking for deep, committed participation in areas that are truly of importance to you. Only then are they able to gain some insights as to your real interests and judge how well your goals and their missions align.

Examples of Experiences Likely to Be Important to Admissions Committees

- Serving as the primary caregiver for an ill family member
- Obstacles or hardships overcome
- Employment history (especially if medically related)
- Research experience
- Experience in a health care setting
- Participation and leadership in community-based or volunteer organizations

Source: Roadmap to Diversity: Integrating Holistic Review into Medical School Admissions Processes, AAMC 2010

serve the needs of their patients, community, and the medical profession at large. They seek a broadly diverse student body because diversity consistently has been shown to drive educational and professional excellence. Schools look for applicants who have developed a track record that demonstrates the knowledge, skills, attitudes, and behaviors that will best prepare them to navigate challenges and thrive as both learners and physicians. Depending upon its mission, one school might look for applicants who demonstrate service to communities underserved by the current health care system, while another may seek applicants who have shown creativity and independent productivity in scholarly activities.

Admissions officers carefully review a multitude of criteria—rather than focusing on just one or two facets—to gain an appreciation of the "whole" person. Many applicants erroneously believe that admissions officers weigh high GPAs and MCAT® scores above all else. While these academic metrics are important components of the admissions decision, they are only one part of the overall package. An applicant's ability to balance multiple priorities and responsibilities as well as the resilience they've shown in handling various issues is considered along with grades and MCAT scores. This helps explain why there are many cases in which a high-scoring student with a near-perfect GPA may not get into medical school and why others with scores and grades below the average do.

More than academic metrics impacts admissions decisions.

Experiences

Your experiences convey a lot about your interests, responsibilities, capabilities, and knowledge. As a result, medical schools take a close look at what you've learned from where you've been up to this stage in your life. It helps them gauge not only how likely you are to be successful in their programs, but also to what degree you will support their mission and contribute as a physician.

The chapter on undergraduate preparation mentioned how important your extracurricular activities may be to an admissions committee. And not just those clubs and organizations within your college, but also outside of school. Your experiences—particularly those related to medicine or research—are an important component that affects your competitiveness as a candidate. For instance, if you are balancing a 20 to 30 hour-a-week job to pay for school while attending classes or have responsibilities caring for a younger sibling or elderly relative, those experiences are important for admissions committees to know about. They communicate information about your different attributes and provide additional context for interpreting your grades. Your experiences—and the insights you gained from them—also help admission committees identify what is unique about you and how you may contribute to their school and the practice of medicine.

Beyond that, the degree to which you contributed and participated in these activities is vital. Medical schools value a demonstration of true commitment, so if you have made a significant contribution or impact on an organization or taken on increasing levels of responsibility, you will want to make that clear to the admissions committee. They are interested not only in what you've done, but how you think those experiences have influenced who you are and what you want to do.

Again, the mission of each school will play a large part in how your experience is evaluated. For example, institutions whose goal is to increase the number of physicians practicing in underserved areas will focus attention on the summer you spent volunteering in a free clinic or rural or urban community outreach on health promotion. In general, medical schools especially value community or volunteer experience related to the health care field.

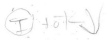

Examples of Attributes Likely to Be Important to Admissions Committees

- Adaptability
- Critical thinking
- Integrity
- Logical reasoning
- Oral communication skills
- Personal maturity
- Reliability
- Self-discipline
- Work habits

- Compassion
- Cultural competence
- Intellectual curiosity
- Motivation for medicine
- Persistence
- Professionalism
- Resilience

Assessing Attributes

Admissions committees use various means and methods to determine if you possess these qualities. While personal experiences such as volunteering for three consecutive summers at a medical clinic certainly conveys dedication and helps demonstrate your proficiency in these areas, admissions committees will look to your personal statement, letters of evaluation, and interview(s) to gauge whether you have the desire to build upon these characteristics in medical school.

Concept of "Distance Traveled"

Here's another thing to consider: admissions officers are likely to place significance on any obstacles or hardships you've overcome to get to this point in your education. This concept, known as "distance traveled," refers to those life challenges you've faced and conquered. Medical schools view these instances as admirable experiences indicative of some very positive traits such as resilience and persistence. As with other experiences, you can help the admissions committee better understand and appreciate your unique contributions by not only describing the experience, but also how these experiences have helped influence you and your desire to be a physician.

Attributes

Admissions committees want to know if you have what it takes to become a competent and compassionate doctor. This includes the ability to master the science and medicine behind it all, of course, but it also requires you to have some key personal attributes.

Are you empathetic? Do you have integrity? Can you communicate effectively and with people different from yourself? Traits such as these are necessary to develop into the kind of physician needed for the future.

Medical schools analyze a broad range of attributes, including those related to the applicant's skills and abilities, personal and professional characteristics, and demographic factors.

- **Skills and abilities** could include active listening, critical thinking, and multilingual ability.

- **Personal and professional characteristics** could include resilience, intellectual curiosity, and empathy.

- **Demographic factors** could include socioeconomic status, race, and gender.

In addition to these general qualities, medical schools give weight to specific characteristics that align with their missions. Examples could include research inquisitiveness, empathy, teamwork, curiosity, and a desire for knowledge about health care delivery systems.

Academic Metrics

Admissions committees need to determine if you have the academic skills and knowledge necessary to succeed in medical school. Committee members will consider your academic record and MCAT scores to answer those questions. Together, these two measures can provide objective information about your knowledge and ability.

Academic History

Your academic history helps admissions committees determine if your study skills, persistence, course of study, and grades predict success at their medical school. Committee members carefully review your college transcript and consider:

- Grades earned in each course and laboratory

- Grade trends in the last two years of schooling

- Number of credit hours carried in each academic period

- Distribution of coursework among the biological, physical, and social sciences, and the humanities

- Need for remediation of unsatisfactory academic work

- Number of incomplete grades and course withdrawals

- Number of years taken to complete the degree program

- The amount of advanced coursework completed in addition to the standard prerequisites and requirements

MCAT Scores

Admissions committees can better predict success when they add MCAT scores into the mix. That's because there can be significant differences in grading scales and standards from college to college, but MCAT scores provide admissions officers with a standardized measure by which to compare applicants. In fact, the ability of admissions officers to predict who will be successful in the first two years of their programs increases by as much as 50 percent (gauging by first- and second-year medical school grades) when they look at MCAT scores in conjunction with undergraduate GPAs as opposed to grades alone.

As a result, the better your grades and higher your scores, the more likely you are to be accepted. It is important to remember that there is still a wide range of MCAT scores and GPAs found among accepted applicants and those are used in conjunction with other factors as discussed earlier in this chapter.

Making the Evaluation

Admissions committees gauge all three of these areas—experiences, attributes, and academic metrics—and how they relate to each other in several ways.

Several elements within the application process speak to your experiences and attributes. Your personal statement, as mentioned in Chapter 6, provides the opportunity for you to tell committee members about your extracurricular activities, distance traveled, volunteer efforts, and medical-related work experience. The personal attributes that accompany these activities can often be inferred. For example, a role as an officer in a school club conveys leadership experience. Working in a medical clinic summer after summer demonstrates motivation for medicine. A long history of volunteering with fundraisers for cancer research suggests teamwork and compassion. Applicants can speak to these experiences in their statements and during interviews to further underscore these connections.

Your letters of evaluation, also described in Chapter 6, attest to your personal attributes. Ask your professors and advisor (and other evaluators) to address your persistence, strong work habits, and self-discipline. (The faculty and administrative staff at your undergraduate school will know how to craft a letter, but for others, you might want to suggest a few key concepts.)

Then there are the academic metrics. As you may know, your academic record is part of your AMCAS application and includes both your college transcript(s) and MCAT scores. From there, committee members can determine whether you have the grades, range of coursework, and the foundation of knowledge they seek in their successful applicants.

Schools consider your experiences, attributes, and academic metrics in combination. Together they give shape to what you, as an applicant, may contribute to their medical school and health care at large. So keep in mind, it's not only about what you did and what you know, but it's also about who you are and what you bring to the learning environment and the medical profession.

The Interview Is Key

If you have been invited to an interview, you should feel confident because you've already impressed your reviewers with your strong personal statement, background, letters of evaluation, and academic history. The interview day gives you a chance to tour the medical school's facility and meet the students, faculty, and staff you may be interacting with for the next several years. Take this opportunity to assess the culture and environment and explore if it might be a good fit for you. Now, you have an opportunity to "shine." Medical schools usually interview three, four, even five times as many applicants as their class size and is why the interview is likely to be the number one determining factor at this phase in the assessment.

The fact that interviews are given at all is a significant distinction of medical schools because some professional schools do not require them. This medical school interview attests to the degree to which admissions officers seek—and medical schools value—qualities and characteristics such as empathy, self-awareness, communication ability, and interpersonal skills that can best be judged in a direct interview situation. You can take a number of steps to ensure you're prepared for it:

- *Know the Basics*

  Whether it's for a new job or for a seat in a medical school's entering class, certain similarities exist in all interviewing situations. A good start would be to review any interviewing books in your school's library or pre-health advisor's office, check to see if your advisor or premed club offers a mock-interview session, search online for tips and interview resources.

- *Know What Type of Interview to Expect*

  It helps to be ready for a number of different interview formats. At some schools, interviews are held with individual admissions committee members; at others, group interviews are the norm. While most interviews are held on the medical school campus, some schools have designated interviewers in different geographic regions to minimize time and expense for applicants. (Information about a school's interview policies and procedures usually is provided to applicants in the initial stages of the selection process.) Check the *Medical School Admission Requirements* website (*www.aamc.org/msar*) to find the type of interviews offered such as one-on-one, panel, or video interviews.

- *Be Comfortable with Different Interviewing Styles*

  You probably have had some experience interviewing for summer and part-time jobs (and possibly for your undergraduate school), so it won't surprise you that interviewers have their own styles and follow different formats. Some follow a structured design, asking questions from a predetermined list and assigning numeric scores to each answer. Others prefer a more free-flowing arrangement and provide the applicant with a greater degree of open input. Still others fall somewhat in the middle.

- *Do Your Research*

  Being able to speak knowledgeably about the medical school shows that you are interested and invested in this particular program. Investigate the school thoroughly by reviewing its profile on the *Medical School Admission Requirements* website (*www.aamc.org/msar*), the school's website, the information packet sent to you, and any articles you can find. Your time is limited, so don't waste it by asking questions already answered on their website, in their materials, or on the *Medical School Admission Requirements* website. Try to talk with current students to get an accurate sense of what the school is like from a student perspective. You will want to impress your interviewer with not only your potential for success, but also your interest in the specific institution. You can demonstrate these qualities through your answers to the interviewer's questions as well as by the questions you ask.

- *Practice*

   Most admissions committee members are experienced interviewers who want to learn about the "real" person you are. Be honest and open during your meeting and do not try to just give the answers you think the interviewer wants to hear. Try to keep the interview conversational. If you're apprehensive about the process, asking a trusted advisor or friend to conduct mock interviews with you can help build your confidence.

   Remember, the interview is an opportunity to discuss your personal history and motivation for pursuing a career in medicine. It also gives you a chance to address any aspects of your application that merit emphasis or explanation. Be sure to present yourself in the best possible light by preparing thoroughly for your meeting. Think about how you conduct yourself among current students and staff during informal meetings, too. Every interaction can create an impression of who you are and how you present yourself may come up during a post-interview discussion.

A Few Last Reminders for When Your Interview Day Arrives

When it comes to what to wear, a good rule of thumb is to dress for the job you seek. In short, look professional. Your interview is likely to be coupled with a tour of the campus, so be sure to wear shoes and an outfit that you are comfortable walking in.

Your interview day is a long one. You will be doing a lot of talking and meeting numerous people. It's okay to bring a water bottle or drink with you. It's very important to be aware that everyone on campus you encounter is someone who potentially can give positive and/or negative feedback about you. Be sure to use good manners, be courteous to all, and show your enthusiasm. Lastly, keep your phone out of sight and on silent. You should not have it out at any time during the interview or campus tour. Remember, they are not only evaluating your academic potential, but also seeing how you conduct yourself professionally, and if you are a good fit for their medical school.

Although interviewers are instructed by admissions officers and guided by federal statutes on what are unfair or discriminatory pre-admission inquiries, there may be an occasion when an interviewer asks an inappropriate question. (See examples in box at right.)

You have the right not to answer what you sense is an inappropriate question. If such a question is asked, try to relax and provide a thoughtful and articulate response (two essential characteristics of a good physician). You also may respectfully decline to answer the question and explain that you were advised not to answer questions that you sensed were inappropriate.

You have the responsibility to report being asked an inappropriate question to help prevent further occurrences. Medical schools have the responsibility to establish procedures that enable applicants to report such incidents in a confidential manner. Medical schools should inform applicants of these procedures prior to interviews and assure them that reporting an incident will not bias the applicant's evaluation.

If a medical school did not inform you of its procedures and an incident occurs, use these guidelines. If possible, report in confidence the interviewer's name and the interview question(s) that was asked to an admissions officer during the interview day. Otherwise, email this information to an admissions officer within 24 hours of the interview noting the date and time of the incident. Furthermore, you have the right to ask if another interview is deemed necessary to ensure an unbiased evaluation of your application to that medical school.

Some interviewers use the interview to assess how well you function under stress and may purposely ask challenging questions to observe how you respond under pressure. How you communicate will be a critical part of the encounter; however, this does not give an interviewer the right to ask you inappropriate questions in their attempt to challenge you during the interview.

Examples of inappropriate questions:

- What is your race, ethnicity, religion, sexual orientation, political affiliation, marital status, opinion on abortion and/or euthanasia, income, value of your home, credit score, etc.?
- Are you planning on having children during medical school?
- Do you have any disabilities?
- Will you require special accommodations?
- Have you ever been arrested?
- Have you ever done drugs?
- How old are you?

Sample responses to inappropriate questions:

Q. *What are your plans for expanding your family during medical school?*

A. Can you please clarify your question? I want to make sure that I'm providing information that is most relevant to my candidacy.

Q. *Have you ever done drugs?*

A. I am uncomfortable discussing my medical history and possible use of prescription medication.

Chapter 8:

Building Toward Greater Diversity

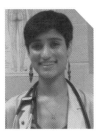

Tehreem Rehman
M.D. Candidate
Yale School of Medicine
Class of 2017

When I met my peers at the beginning of medical school, the breadth of their experiences amazed me. It was humbling. My preconceptions were challenged. While our diverse backgrounds were a fascinating point of discussion, many of their experiences also provided new perspectives on health care issues such as mistrust of providers, language barriers, and structural causes of health inequity.

As research studies have proven, the educational experience is enhanced when the student body includes individuals from varying cultures and backgrounds. Diversity generates a wealth of ideas, helps students challenge their assumptions, and broadens their perspectives. The AAMC strives to increase diversity among medical school applicants, and many medical schools offer programs to ensure that all candidates have an equal opportunity for admittance. In fact, in my own situation, if it weren't for a merit-based scholarship for disadvantaged students, I would not have been able to attend my current school. Promoting diversity also means recognizing unequal playing fields that exist in our society and, subsequently, extending opportunities to disenfranchised but capable individuals.

My own experience, as a low-income first-generation college student and a Muslim woman of color played pivotal roles in my desire to pursue a career in medicine. I believe that physicians have a social responsibility to advocate for the needs of the communities they serve. Despite the fact that poverty is pervasive and this nation has great racial/ethnic diversity, when I began medical school, I recognized that our courses lacked information on how health inequities disproportionately impact low-income Americans and those of color. In response, a classmate and I developed a course, U.S. Health Justice, to help students identify health disparities in this country and gain advocacy skills to create change.

Diversity in group settings even has been linked to greater intellectual results, ultimately leading to better learning outcomes. Alongside learning about organ systems and diseases in the classroom, students truly can benefit from the insight of their peers; however, such insight is only possible by ensuring that historically marginalized communities are represented in the cohort of the next generation of physicians in training.

Defining Diversity

What exactly is meant by "diversity?"

When you hear the word diversity, many people automatically think in terms of race and ethnicity. And while it is certainly important to have more racial and ethnic minority populations represented in medicine, the concept of diversity is much more expansive. Diversity refers to the richness of human differences—socioeconomic status, race, ethnicity, language, nationality, sex, gender identity, sexual orientation, religion, geography, disability, age, and individual aspects such as personality, learning styles, and life experiences. Let's look at diversity based on available AAMC data and other information.

- **First, consider race and ethnicity.** While diversity extends beyond this particular characteristic, it remains a critical component. The data show, for example, that only 6.1 percent of matriculating students are black or African-American, 9.2 percent are Hispanic or Latino, and 0.3 percent are American Indian or Alaska Native.

- **What about family income?** This is another area of great imbalance. Parental income of students entering medical school skews heavily to the upper range, with median income of $120,000. (That's almost double the estimated U.S. median family income of $52,100 reported by the U.S. Census Bureau.) Looking at it from another angle, almost one in six students comes from a home in which their parents earn $250,000 or more a year.

- **Another perspective—gender.** On the surface, it appears that male and female applicants are fairly equal in number, but there are instances where that is not the case. You will see, for example, in chart 8-A, there is a relative shortage of male applicants within the black or African-American demographic. Within this specific group, males comprise barely one-third of those who apply to medical school.

AAMC Programs and Resources

The AAMC is strongly committed to improving health for all. Considering all of the benefits that diversity offers (outlined throughout this chapter), the AAMC is engaged in a number of programs and initiatives designed to help increase diversity to include all capable and promising students from a broad range of backgrounds. While these programs are open to all students, they are sensitive to the challenges and needs of individuals from groups underrepresented in medicine. These initiatives are described below.

Career Fairs and Enrichment Programs

Medical schools throughout the country provide various programs and resources designed to recruit students and prepare them for medical education. Some of these programs are held during the school year, others in the summer. They are designed for high school students, college students, and those who already have completed undergraduate study.

The AAMC is affiliated with two such programs:

- ***Minority Student Medical Career Awareness Workshops and Recruitment Fair***
  This event typically is held each fall in conjunction with Learn Serve Lead: The AAMC Annual Meeting. Students are encouraged to come and explore the possibilities in medicine. College and high school students, parents, pre-health advisors, school administrators, and any others interested in pursuing a career in medicine can meet diversity affairs and admissions officers from U.S. medical schools and other health professions schools to discuss medical school preparation, enrichment programs, admissions policies and procedures, financial aid, and more. Attendees also can participate in interactive medical and health activities and workshops. For more information, visit *www.aamc.org/medicalcareerfair.*

- ***Summer Medical and Dental Education Program (SMDEP)***
  The Summer Medical and Dental Education Program is a free six-week academic enrichment program for college freshmen and sophomores interested in careers in medicine or dentistry. Components of the program include science- and mathematics-based courses, learning and study skills seminars, career development activities, clinical experiences, and a financial planning workshop. Funded by the Robert Wood Johnson Foundation and offered at 12 U.S. medical and nine dental schools across the nation, the program includes a stipend, housing, and meals. For additional information, visit *www.smdep.org,* or call toll free at 1-866-58SMDEP.

Low-Income Households Are Underrepresented…

Parental Income of Entering Medical Students, 2013

Income	Percent
Less than $25,000	6.7
$25,000 – $49,999	8.4
$50,000 – $74,999	11.2
$75,000 – $99,999	10.0
$100,000 – $149,999	19.3
$150,000 – $199,999	12.4
$200,000 – $249,999	10.3
$250,000 – $299,999	5.03
$300,000 – $399,999	6.3
$400,000 – $499,999	3.7
$500,000 or more	6.6
Median income of parents	$120,000

Source: AAMC's 2014 Matriculating Student Questionnaire (MSQ)

Racial Ethnic Minorities Are Underrepresented…

Demographics of Entering Medical Students*, 2014

Demographic	Percent
American Indian or Alaska Native	0.2
Hispanic/Latino	6.0
Black or African-American	6.0
Asian	19.0
White	52.1

self-identified. Source: AAMC Data Warehouse, 2014

Aspiring Docs—An AAMC Program to Increase Diversity in Medicine

It is vital for tomorrow's medical students to be diverse in terms of race, ethnicity, gender, religion, socioeconomic status, and sexual orientation, as well as express diversity through their experiences and thoughts. Having a diverse workforce of doctors is essential to providing the best care for all communities and improving the health of all.

Aspiring Docs offers the most reliable tools and information to anyone considering a career in medicine. To access the growing library of information and resources, visit *www.aamc.org/aspiringdocs.*

Chart 8-A

Applicants to U.S. Medical Schools by Race, Ethnicity, and Sex, 2013**

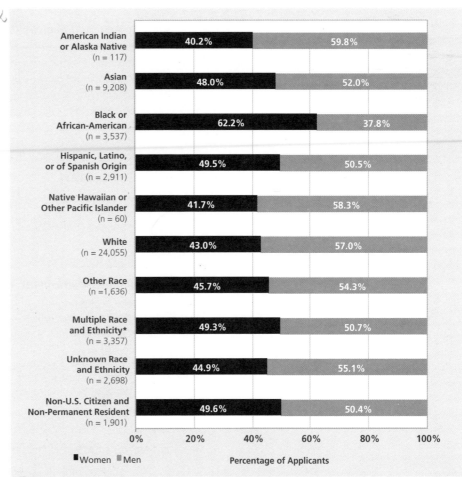

Note:
* = Six applicants in 2014 who declined to report gender are not reflected.
** = Multiple Race/Ethnicity includes those who indicated more than one race or ethnicity category (e.g., "Black or African-American" and "American Indian or Alaska Native", "Hispanic, Latino, or of Spanish Origin"and "White").
Source: AAMC public website: https://www.aamc.org/download/321480/data/factstable12.pdf

Additional AAMC Resources

The AAMC also offers a wide variety of publications, online tools, and other information in the AAMC's Minorities in Medicine website at *www.aamc.org/students/minorities*, and the Diversity and Inclusion website at *www.aamc.org/diversity*. Among the resources you will find are:

- ### *Medical Students with Disabilities: Resources to Enhance Accessibility*
  This recently published guide informs users about current resources available to medical schools as they accept and matriculate a growing number of medical students with a wide range of disabilities. Specifically, there is an emphasis in this publication on the assistive technologies available for medical students. You can order a copy of this guide at *https://members.aamc.org/eweb/DynamicPage.aspx?webcode=PubHome*.

- ### *Enrichment Programs Online*
  This site includes a free database to help students locate summer enrichment programs on medical school campuses. You can search by school, state, region, area of focus, and length of program. Go to *https://services.aamc.org/summerprograms/* to explore programs of interest.

- ### *Medical Minority Applicant Registry (Med-MAR)*
  During the MCAT registration, students who are either economically disadvantaged or from racial and ethnic groups that are historically underrepresented in medicine can select the Medical Minority Applicant Registry (Med-MAR) option to be included in the registry. This web-based program provides medical schools with basic biographical information and MCAT scores of registered examinees, thereby providing institutions with opportunities to enhance their diversity efforts. Go to *www.aamc.org/medmar* for more information.

  For information about the definition of underrepresented in medicine, visit *www.aamc.org/urm*.

- ### *Fee Assistance Program (FAP)*
  The AAMC believes that the cost of applying to medical school should not be an insurmountable barrier and offers a Fee Assistance Program (FAP), which is available to students whose financial limitations would otherwise prevent them from taking the MCAT exam or applying to medical school. Details about FAP can be found at *https://www.aamc.org/students/applying/fap/* and in Chapter 6 of this book.

- ### *Data About Applicants, Matriculants, and Graduates*
  The AAMC also collects and presents detailed data about medical students from different racial and ethnic groups, most of which are available online free of charge on the AAMC website (and a good deal of which is included in this guide). Several resources likely to be of interest are:

  — AAMC information about recent matriculant data for each medical school is presented in this chapter in Table 8-A, Matriculants by Medical School and Self-Identification, 2014.

  — Chapter 10 includes a table showing the self-identification of medical school applicants and accepted applicants for the 2014 entering class.

  — A large collection of data about medical school applicants, matriculants, and graduates is available on the AAMC website at *www.aamc.org/facts*.

  — The AAMC publication, *Diversity in Medical Education, Facts & Figures 2014*, provides race and ethnicity data on medical school applicants, accepted applicants, matriculants, enrollment, graduates, and faculty. You can access the full text without charge at *http://aamcdiversityfactsandfigures.org*.

  — Data on medical school faculty, including information by self-identification, can be found at *www.aamc.org/data/facultyroster/reports*.

For those who wish to explore the benefits of diversity, may we suggest the following readings:

Antonio AL, Chang MJ, Hakuta K, Kenny DA, Levin S, Milem JF. Effects of racial diversity on complex thinking in college students. *Psychological Science*. 2004:15;507–10.

Astin AW. *What matters in college? Four critical years revisited*. San Francisco, CA: Jossey-Bass; 1993.

Gurin P. *The compelling need for diversity in higher education: Expert testimony in Gratz, et al. v. Bollinger, et al.* Michigan J of Race & Law. 1999:5;363–425.

Nemeth CJ, Wachtler J. Creative problem solving as a result of majority vs. minority influence. *European J of Social Psychology*. 1983:13;45–55.

Nivet MA. Commentary: Diversity 3.0: A necessary systems upgrade. *Acad Med*. 2011;86:1487–1489.

Saha S, Guiton G, Wimmers PF, Wilkerson L. *Student body racial and ethnic composition and diversity-related outcomes in US medical schools*. JAMA. 2008:300:1135–1145.

Smith DG & Associates. *Diversity works: The emerging picture of how students benefit*. Washington, DC: Association of American Colleges and Universities; 1997.

Smith DG. *Diversity's Promise for Higher Education: Making It Work*. Baltimore, M.D.: The Johns Hopkins University Press; 2009.

Whitla, DK, Orfield G, Silen W, Teperow C, Howard C, & Reede J. (2003). Educational benefits of diversity in medical school: A survey of students. Acad Med. 2003;78:460–466.

School Programs and Resources

Just as the AAMC is committed to the issue of diversity, colleges and medical schools also are invested in making medical education accessible to all. Take some time to explore these resources as well:

- **Premedical School Programs at Undergraduate Colleges**
  Pre-health advisors have an abundance of information and data at their fingertips. Not only can they help you with the application process and refer you to appropriate contacts, they also know about programs that students from underrepresented groups and disadvantaged backgrounds have found useful. If your college has a pre-health advisor (and the majority of them do), make sure you take advantage of this valuable resource. Learn more about pre-health advisors or to locate one if your school does not have an advising office, visit *www.naahp.org*.

- **Medical School Websites**
  In addition to the individual profiles in the *Medical School Admission Requirements* website, you'll also want to explore the medical school websites for information on their diversity programs and resources. Go to *www.aamc.org/medicalschools* for a listing of all U.S. and Canadian M.D.-granting medical schools and links to their websites.

- **Medical School Diversity Affairs Representatives**
  Another invaluable resource is medical school diversity affairs representatives. These individuals are dedicated to increasing diversity among medical schools at their institutions and are an excellent source of information for applicants (or potential applicants). You can get the name of the diversity affairs contacts at any U.S. medical school through the Directory of Diversity Affairs Representatives searchable database. It is searchable by name, location, and institution, and is available at *www.aamc.org/coda*. Contact information also is available within each medical school profile on the *Medical School Admission Requirements* website at *www.aamc.org/msar*.

- **Financial Assistance for Medical School**
  Don't let the cost of medical school deter you from your dreams. As you will learn in Chapter 11, more than four-fifths of medical students across the country receive some form of financial assistance. Medical schools—both public and private—work hard to offer a variety of financial aid plans to ensure that capable students are not denied access to their institutions as a result of financial limitations. In addition to discussing possibilities for assistance with the financial aid officer at the medical schools that interest you, you should familiarize yourself with general information about financing a medical education by reading the relevant material in this book and reviewing the wealth of information about loans (and other programs) at *www.aamc.org/first*.

- **Programs at Medical Schools**
  Once you've enrolled in medical school, you will find that a variety of academic and personal support programs are available to you. These programs help students from various backgrounds to successfully complete their medical studies, with the ultimate goal of increasing diversity among physicians entering careers in patient care, teaching, and research, and eliminating racial and ethnic disparities in health care.

No Advisor? Contact the NAAHP for Help

If your institution does not have a pre-health advisor, you can contact the National Association of Advisors for the Health Professions (NAAHP). There, you will find a list of NAAHP members who have volunteered to help students without access to a pre-health advisor from a distance. Learn more about what pre-health advisors do and how to locate one at *www.naahp.org/StudentResources/FindanAdvisor.aspx*.

Table 8-A:

Matriculants by Medical School and Race and Ethnicity, 2014*

State	School	Hispanic or Latino	Asian	Native American (incl AK)	Black	Native Hawaiian/ OPI	White	Other	Unduplicated Total
AL	Alabama	5	29	2	10	1	137	5	186
AL	South Alabama	0	9	0	8	1	55	4	76
AR	Arkansas	6	14	3	7	1	137	5	168
AZ	Arizona	10	24	3	2	0	67	12	115
AZ	Arizona Phoenix	9	12	3	3	1	49	7	80
CA	Loma Linda	14	60	4	16	3	72	6	168
CA	Southern Cal-Keck	11	71	1	12	0	64	11	185
CA	Stanford	8	35	1	6	0	34	5	90
CA	UC Berkeley/SF Joint Prog	3	7	2	0	0	9	0	16
CA	UC Davis	30	33	0	7	1	30	7	110
CA	UC Irvine	11	33	1	1	1	50	12	104
CA	UC Riverside	7	21	0	3	0	14	7	50
CA	UC San Diego	19	43	1	10	1	52	6	124
CA	UC San Francisco	22	50	3	21	1	58	5	149
CA	UCLA Drew	11	1	0	14	0	0	0	24
CA	UCLA-Geffen	16	50	3	18	1	50	9	151
CO	Colorado	27	34	4	8	1	112	7	182
CT	Connecticut	7	20	3	15	0	62	1	98
CT	Quinnipiac-Netter	3	23	0	0	0	57	6	90
CT	Yale	5	32	1	7	0	42	5	104
DC	George Washington	16	40	2	14	1	87	8	178
DC	Georgetown	4	25	2	12	0	139	8	196
DC	Howard	14	15	0	72	0	7	7	117
FL	FIU-Wertheim	42	22	0	12	0	53	6	119
FL	Florida	16	15	1	19	0	90	7	135
FL	Florida Atlantic-Schmidt	5	11	0	1	0	41	4	64
FL	Florida State	20	12	2	16	0	66	8	120
FL	Miami-Miller	18	47	0	7	0	116	15	199
FL	UCF	11	31	2	1	1	67	14	120
FL	USF-Morsani	13	49	1	6	0	96	8	170
GA	Emory	7	25	1	9	0	84	9	135
GA	GRU MC Georgia	15	40	1	25	0	141	5	230
GA	Mercer	2	12	0	4	0	82	4	107
GA	Morehouse	6	7	0	52	1	8	3	78
HI	Hawaii-Burns	0	54	0	0	7	15	1	66
IA	Iowa-Carver	8	24	2	3	1	113	4	152
IL	Chicago Med Franklin	15	54	1	10	2	86	11	190
IL	Chicago-Pritzker	7	17	2	11	0	56	2	90
IL	Illinois	50	79	3	23	0	141	10	297
IL	Loyola-Stritch	19	18	1	13	0	102	8	161
IL	Northwestern-Feinberg	17	52	2	4	0	72	1	163
IL	Rush	7	29	0	11	1	71	2	128
IL	Southern Illinois	1	6	0	6	0	58	0	72
IN	Indiana	32	51	4	32	0	228	12	352
KS	Kansas	17	15	7	11	1	175	7	211
KY	Kentucky	3	13	0	3	0	103	5	136
KY	Louisville	1	13	3	15	0	124	4	157
LA	LSU New Orleans	8	24	0	13	0	146	4	194
LA	LSU Shreveport	3	10	2	4	0	102	4	123
LA	Tulane	10	41	0	7	0	122	8	198
MA	Boston	27	45	1	5	1	82	9	166
MA	Harvard	17	50	2	11	1	61	5	164
MA	Massachusetts	3	24	1	2	0	84	4	125
MA	Tufts	8	43	3	10	2	125	9	200
MD	Johns Hopkins	11	37	1	5	0	57	5	118
MD	Maryland	4	41	1	8	0	94	5	157
MD	Uniformed Services-Hebert	13	26	2	7	1	126	7	173
MI	Central Michigan	1	11	0	0	0	80	10	104
MI	Michigan	10	38	2	10	1	113	4	176
MI	Michigan State	17	24	3	23	1	110	11	190
MI	Oakland Beaumont	2	31	3	6	1	49	10	100
MI	Wayne State	2	56	1	5	0	162	17	290
MI	Western Michigan	1	15	3	1	0	31	5	54

Source: AAMC Data Warehouse Applicants as of 10/29/2014
* Data is not reflective of the number of individuals in each demographic category, but the number of times a particular racial or ethnic category was selected. One individual can self-identify with multiple groups.

Table 8-A:

Matriculants by Medical School and Race and Ethnicity, 2014* (continued)

State	School	Hispanic or Latino	Asian	Native American (incl AK)	Black	Native Hawaiian/ OPI	White	Other	Unduplicated Total
MN	Mayo	2	11	1	4	0	33	0	53
MN	Minnesota	15	20	5	17	0	169	5	230
MO	Missouri Columbia	1	7	0	1	0	92	2	104
MO	Missouri Kansas City	4	49	2	10	0	46	1	121
MO	Saint Louis	4	56	0	7	1	100	7	180
MO	Washington U St Louis	10	38	1	6	0	64	4	123
MS	Mississippi	1	16	3	14	0	111	2	145
NC	Duke	4	26	1	16	1	57	1	109
NC	East Carolina-Brody	2	7	1	8	0	55	3	80
NC	North Carolina	12	26	2	26	0	115	5	180
NC	Wake Forest	3	18	1	8	0	85	3	120
ND	North Dakota	0	1	7	1	0	70	2	78
NE	Creighton	6	29	0	8	0	111	3	155
NE	Nebraska	6	10	1	2	0	110	2	128
NH	Dartmouth-Geisel	14	22	1	8	1	35	4	89
NJ	Cooper Rowan	4	8	2	9	0	46	2	72
NJ	Rutgers New Jersey	30	73	0	18	0	56	12	178
NJ	Rutgers-RW Johnson	4	41	1	11	0	76	5	142
NM	New Mexico	28	13	6	5	1	51	6	103
NV	Nevada	5	17	0	2	1	46	2	70
NY	Albany	12	40	0	6	0	73	7	138
NY	Buffalo	21	24	1	5	0	92	4	144
NY	Columbia	20	27	0	17	1	87	5	157
NY	Cornell-Weill	6	24	2	10	0	55	5	101
NY	Hofstra North Shore-LIJ	12	29	0	7	0	49	2	98
NY	Mount Sinai-Icahn	13	38	0	12	0	67	4	140
NY	New York Medical	25	35	0	14	0	106	12	196
NY	New York University	10	50	1	3	1	75	6	149
NY	Rochester	8	28	0	9	0	48	1	102
NY	SUNY Downstate	11	56	0	14	0	81	7	188
NY	SUNY Upstate	5	29	0	10	0	92	3	154
NY	Stony Brook	9	42	0	7	0	59	4	128
NY	Yeshiva Einstein	10	43	0	6	0	103	7	183
OH	Case Western Reserve	13	64	0	7	0	100	4	207
OH	Cincinnati	9	43	1	11	1	93	8	171
OH	Northeast Ohio	3	39	2	3	0	91	9	147
OH	Ohio State	18	45	2	16	1	113	5	192
OH	Toledo	2	34	0	7	0	115	12	176
OH	Wright State-Boonshoft	7	15	1	19	1	66	5	108
OK	Oklahoma	5	29	14	3	0	122	6	165
OR	Oregon	7	23	3	1	3	93	10	139
PA	Commonwealth	9	12	0	3	0	72	5	100
PA	Drexel	10	88	3	21	0	122	14	260
PA	Jefferson-Kimmel	17	43	3	4	0	173	1	260
PA	Penn State	6	24	0	0	1	111	3	148
PA	Pennsylvania-Perelman	26	39	0	12	2	86	2	157
PA	Pittsburgh	7	48	0	11	0	66	8	147
PA	Temple	12	50	1	10	0	156	7	232
PR	Caribe	60	1	0	0	0	14	0	65
PR	Ponce	67	1	0	1	0	11	1	70
PR	Puerto Rico	110	2	0	1	0	9	1	110
PR	San Juan Bautista	54	1	0	1	0	4	5	63
RI	Brown-Alpert	12	42	0	18	1	49	1	125
SC	MU South Carolina	8	11	0	24	0	130	3	176
SC	South Carolina	3	15	0	6	0	64	1	96
SC	South Carolina Greenville	8	3	1	7	0	64	2	82
SD	South Dakota-Sanford	0	3	0	0	0	54	0	58
TN	East Tennessee-Quillen	1	5	0	0	0	63	2	72
TN	Meharry	13	10	3	68	1	12	0	105
TN	Tennessee	6	19	0	18	1	114	0	165
TN	Vanderbilt	9	18	1	6	2	48	3	88

Source: AAMC Data Warehouse Applicants as of 10/29/2014
* Data is not reflective of the number of individuals in each demographic category, but the number of times a particular racial or ethnic category was selected. One individual can self-identify with multiple groups.

Table 8-A:
Matriculants by Medical School and Race and Ethnicity, 2014* (continued)

State	School	Hispanic or Latino	Asian	Native American (incl AK)	Black	Native Hawaiian/ OPI	White	Other	Unduplicated Total
TX	Baylor	13	71	2	6	0	91	3	185
TX	Texas A & M	19	72	1	9	0	105	2	200
TX	Texas Tech	21	51	4	4	0	108	2	181
TX	Texas Tech-Foster	32	20	0	1	0	59	1	104
TX	UT HSC San Antonio	43	24	2	13	1	145	2	213
TX	UT Houston	47	55	4	20	0	145	4	240
TX	UT Medical Branch	42	65	3	22	1	112	4	231
TX	UT Southwestern	12	85	0	10	1	127	6	232
UT	Utah	2	20	0	0	0	77	2	102
VA	Eastern Virginia	4	39	1	12	1	86	6	150
VA	Virginia	20	33	2	23	1	79	2	156
VA	Virginia Commonwealth	11	61	0	11	1	122	13	216
VA	Virginia Tech Carilion	3	14	1	1	0	21	2	42
VT	Vermont	7	25	0	1	0	74	5	115
WA	U Washington	11	37	3	3	2	180	11	240
WI	MC Wisconsin	16	33	4	10	5	131	4	204
WI	Wisconsin	3	23	4	4	0	128	5	176
WV	Marshall-Edwards	3	6	0	2	0	63	6	79
WV	West Virginia	4	12	0	4	0	88	1	110

Source: AAMC Data Warehouse Applicants as of 10/29/2014
* Data is not reflective of the number of individuals in each demographic category, but the number of times a particular racial or ethnic category was selected. One individual can self-identify with multiple groups.

Chapter 9:

Be in the Know: Application and Acceptance Protocols—Admissions Officers

These recommendations correspond directly with the AAMC Recommendations for Applicants in Chapter 6

The AAMC recommends the following guidelines to ensure that M.D. and M.D.-Ph.D. applicants are afforded timely notification of the outcome of their applications, have timely access to available first-year positions, and that schools and programs are protected from having unfilled positions in their entering classes. These protocols are often referred to as "traffic rules" by admissions officers and pre-health advisors. These recommendations are distributed to prospective M.D. and M.D.-Ph.D. students, their advisors, and personnel at the medical schools and programs to which they have applied.

The AAMC recommends that each M.D. or M.D.-Ph.D. granting school or program:

1. Comply with established procedures to:

    a. Annually publish, amend, and adhere to its application, acceptance, and admission procedures.

    b. Abide by all conditions of participation agreements with application services (if using).

2. Promptly communicate admissions decisions:

    a. By October 1, notify Early Decision applicants and the American Medical College Application Service® (AMCAS®) of Early Decision Program (EDP) admission actions.

    b. From October 15 to March 15, notify AMCAS within five business days of all admission actions, either written or verbal, that have been communicated to an applicant.

    c. From March 16 to the first day of class, notify AMCAS within two business days of all admissions acceptance, withdrawal, or deferral actions, either written or verbal, that have been communicated to an applicant. All admission actions are listed and defined on the AAMC website.

    d. An acceptance offer is defined as the point at which a medical school communicates a written or verbal acceptance offer to an applicant.

    e. An acceptance offer to any dual degree program that occurs after an initial acceptance should follow the above timelines.

3. Notify all regular M.D. program applicants of their acceptance on or after October 15* of each admission cycle, but no earlier. Schools and programs may notify applicants of admissions decisions other than acceptance prior to October 15.

continued...

4. By March 15 of the matriculation year, issue a number of acceptance offers at least equal to the expected number of students in its first-year entering class and report those acceptance actions to AMCAS.

5. On or before April 30, permit **ALL** applicants (except for EDP applicants):

   a. A minimum of two weeks to respond to their acceptance offer.

   b. To hold acceptance offers or a waitlist position from any other schools or programs without penalty (i.e., scholarships).

6. After April 30, implement school-specific procedures for accepted applicants who, without adequate explanation, continue to hold one or more places at other schools or programs.

   a. Each school or program should permit applicants:

      1. A minimum of five business days to respond to an acceptance offer. This may be reduced to a minimum of two business days within 30 days of the start of orientation.

      2. Submit a statement of intent, a deposit, or both.

   b. Recognize the challenges of applicants with multiple acceptance offers, applicants who have not yet received an acceptance offer, and applicants who have not yet been informed about financial aid opportunities at schools to which they have been accepted.

   c. Permit applicants who have been accepted or who have been granted a deferral, to remain on other schools' or programs' wait lists. Also, permit these applicants to withdraw if they later receive an acceptance offer from a preferred school or program.

7. Each school's pre-enrollment deposit should not exceed $100 and (except for EDP applicants,) be refundable until April 30. If the applicant enrolls at the school, the school should credit the deposit toward tuition. Schools should not require additional deposits or matriculation fees prior to matriculation.

8. On or after May 15, any school that plans to make an acceptance offer to an applicant who has already been accepted to, or granted a deferral by, another school or program, must ensure that the other school or program is advised of this offer at the time it is issued (written or verbal) to the applicant. This notification should be made **immediately by telephone and email** by the close of business on the same day. The communication should contain the applicants name and AAMC ID number, the program being offered (e.g., M.D. only, joint program), and the date through which the offer is valid. Schools and programs should communicate fully with each other with respect to anticipated late roster changes in order to minimize inter-school miscommunication and misunderstanding, as well as to prevent unintended vacant positions in a school's first-year entering class.

9. No school or program should make an acceptance offer, either verbal or written, to any individual who has officially matriculated/enrolled in, or begun an orientation program immediately prior to enrollment at an LCME accredited medical school. Medical programs should enter a matriculation action for students in AMCAS immediately upon the start of enrollment or the orientation immediately preceding enrollment.

10. Each school should treat all letters of evaluation submitted in support of an application as **confidential**, except in those states with applicable laws to the contrary. The contents of a letter of evaluation should not be revealed to an applicant at any time.

*If any date falls on a weekend/holiday the recommendation(s) will apply to the following business day.

Approved: AAMC Committee on Admissions, September 2014

Chapter 10:

Applicant and Acceptee Data

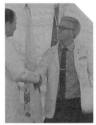

Luke P. Burns
M.D. Candidate
University of California,
San Diego, School
of Medicine
Class of 2018

When applying to medical school, it's difficult not to transform yourself into a number—well, two numbers: your MCAT score and GPA. While these figures will determine part of your success in applying to medical school, they are only two facets of a far more complex tapestry you eventually will weave.

I often found myself riddled with self-doubt during that difficult "glide year" between applying [to school] and matriculation. Was my MCAT score high enough? Should I have retaken it? Would admissions committees overlook that low grade in a science class or that summer I should have spent doing research? It would always take a conversation with a family member, close friend, or mentor to remind me that I was more than just a mathematical index on a percentile chart. I was an enthusiastic applicant and a lover of people, and I had plenty of clinical experiences and medical exposure to prove it.

Applying to medical school is a constant assault on your self-esteem as you strive to meet the high standards that many people—but particularly you—set for yourself. Be realistic, but don't be ruthless. Know your weaknesses, but celebrate your strengths. The skills you develop before medical school will inform you for the rest of your life. Those numbers that got you there? They never matter again.

A Quick Look at the 2014 Entering Class

- In 2013–14, 49,480 people applied to the 2014 entering class at all M.D.-granting medical schools in the United States.

- By the fall of 2014, 21,355 applicants had been offered an acceptance to at least one medical school, and 20,343 accepted applicants had matriculated.

These accepted applicants possessed a broad range of MCAT scores and undergraduate GPAs, and a wide variety of personal characteristics and life experiences. Both male and female applicants were distributed across numerous racial and ethnic groups. A small number applied through the Early Decision Program, but the majority used the regular application process. A small number of accepted applicants chose not to matriculate in 2014.

This chapter contains graphic representations of relevant data for the entire applicant pool, as well as for accepted and non-accepted applicants for the 2014 entering class. All data presented in this chapter are accurate as of October 29, 2014*. In the following charts:

- "All applicants" refers to all applicants to the 2014 entering class

- "Accepted applicants" refers to those applicants accepted to at least one medical school

- "Non-accepted applicants" refers to those applicants not accepted to any medical school

In the following pages, we provide data related to performance on the MCAT® exam, undergraduate grade point average (GPA), MCAT scores and undergraduate GPA combined, undergraduate major, gender, age, type of application, and race and ethnicity.

Source: AAMC DataWarehouse; Applicant Matriculant File

Performance on the MCAT exam

Charts 10-A – 10-D present information about the performance of applicants on the MCAT exam:

- **Chart 10-A** shows that applicants achieved Verbal Reasoning (VR) scores at each score from 1 to 15; the largest number achieved a VR score of 10. Accepted applicants' scores ranged from 2 to 15, although very few had VR scores below 5 (just over 50). At a VR score of 11, the number of accepted applicants exceeded the number not accepted.

- **Chart 10-B** shows that applicants achieved Physical Sciences (PS) scores at each score from 1 to 15; the largest number achieved a PS score of 10. Accepted applicants' scores ranged from 1 to 15; about 25 accepted applicants achieved a score of 5 or below. Accepted applicants exceeded non-accepted applicants at a PS score of 11.

Chart 10-A

MCAT® Verbal Reasoning Score Distribution, Year 2014 Applicants

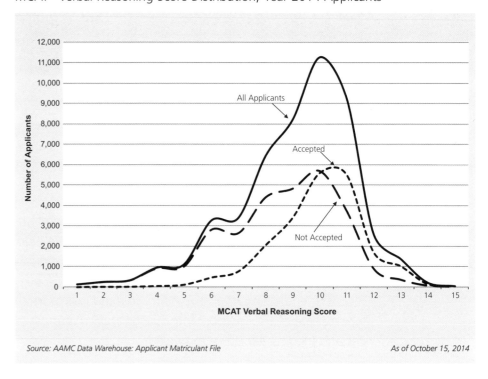

Source: AAMC Data Warehouse: Applicant Matriculant File · As of October 15, 2014

Chart 10-B

MCAT® Physical Sciences Score Distribution, Year 2014 Applicants

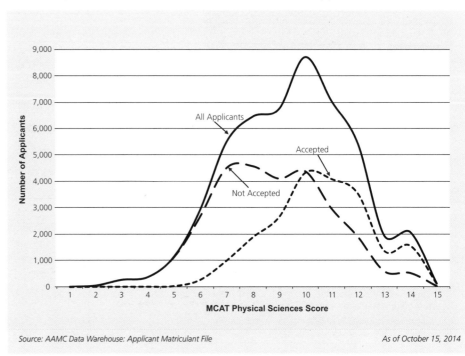

Source: AAMC Data Warehouse: Applicant Matriculant File · As of October 15, 2014

Chart 10-C

MCAT® Biological Sciences Score Distribution, Year 2014 Applicants

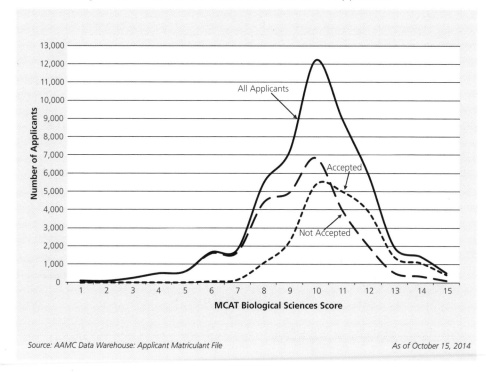

Source: AAMC Data Warehouse: Applicant Matriculant File

As of October 15, 2014

- **Chart 10-C** shows that applicants achieved Biological Sciences (BS) scores at each score from 1 to 15; the largest number achieved a BS score of 10. Accepted applicants' scores ranged from 1 to 15; about 10 scored 5 or below. Accepted applicants exceeded non-accepted applicants at a score of 11.

- **Chart 10-D**—which shows total scores on the numerically scored sections of Verbal Reasoning, Physical Sciences, and Biological Sciences—reveals that applicants achieved total scores from 4 to 54; the largest number achieved a total score of 30. Accepted applicants achieved total scores ranging from 9 to 45; the number of accepted applicants with total scores of 17 and below (an average of almost 6 on each section) was just under 10. Accepted applicants exceeded non-accepted applicants at a total score of 31.

No score on a single MCAT section and no total MCAT score "guarantees" admission to medical school. Charts 10-A, 10-B, and 10-C reveal that, while applicants with VR, PS, and BS scores of 11 and above had a higher probability of being accepted into medical school, a significant number of applicants with such scores were not accepted. Finally, Chart 10-D shows that a substantial number of applicants with total MCAT scores of 30 and above were not accepted. These findings reveal the importance of factors other than MCAT performance—including undergraduate academic performance and a variety of personal characteristics and experiential variables—in the medical student selection process.

Chart 10-D

MCAT® Total Numeric Score Distribution, Year 2014 Applicants

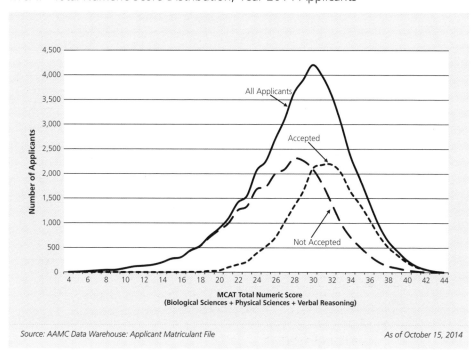

Source: AAMC Data Warehouse: Applicant Matriculant File

As of October 15, 2014

Undergraduate Grade Point Average (GPA)

Charts 10-E—10-G present information about the undergraduate academic performance of applicants:

- **Chart 10-E:** Undergraduate science GPA (biology, chemistry, physics, and mathematics)

- **Chart 10-F:** Undergraduate nonscience GPA

- **Chart 10-G:** Undergraduate total GPA

Chart 10-E shows that the undergraduate science GPAs of all applicants were on a continuum from just under 2.0 to 4.0, on a 4.0 scale; most were between 3.75 and 4.0. Accepted applicants also had undergraduate science GPAs across the entire range, but few had GPAs of 2.50 or below (just over 90). The undergraduate science GPA at which accepted applicants exceeded those not accepted was between 3.50 and 3.75.

Chart 10-F shows applicants' undergraduate nonscience GPAs along the continuum from just under 2.0 to 4.0, with most between 3.75 and 4.0. Accepted applicants' undergraduate nonscience GPAs also ranged from 2.0 to 4.0, but just more than 100 had a GPA of 2.75 or below. At 3.75 to 4.0, accepted applicants exceeded non-accepted applicants.

Chart 10-E

GPA Science Distribution, Year 2014 Applicants

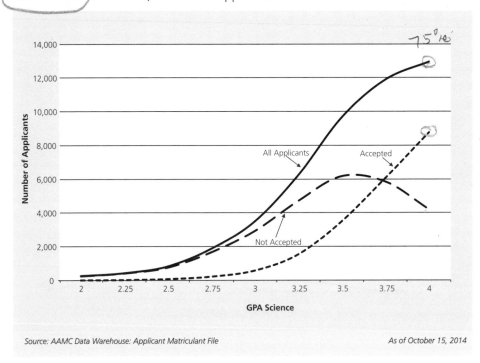

Source: AAMC Data Warehouse: Applicant Matriculant File

As of October 15, 2014

Chart 10-F

GPA Nonscience Distribution, Year 2014 Applicants

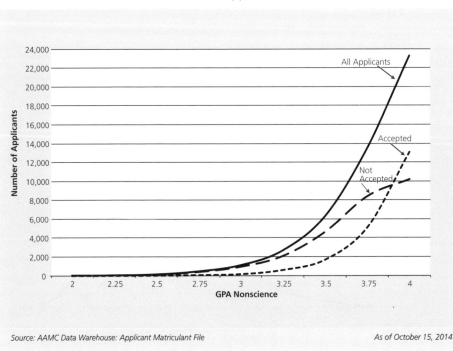

Source: AAMC Data Warehouse: Applicant Matriculant File

As of October 15, 2014

Chart 10-G

GPA Total Distribution, Year 2014 Applicants

2/3 Accepted
1/3 not accep?

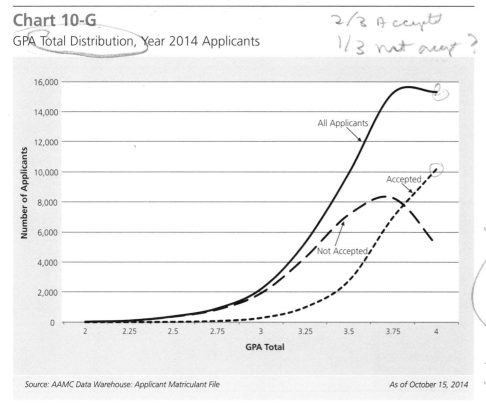

As shown in **Chart 10-G**, all applicants had total undergraduate GPAs from just under 2.0 to 4.0, and most were in the range of 3.75 to 4.0. Accepted applicants' total undergraduate GPAs ranged from just under 2.25 to 4.0, but just about 100 possessed undergraduate total GPAs of 2.75 or below. Accepted applicants exceeded non-accepted applicants at an undergraduate total GPA of between 3.75 and 4.0.

As is the case with MCAT data, GPA data in Charts 10-E–10-G show that no undergraduate GPA ensures admission to medical school. While applicants with undergraduate science, nonscience, and total GPAs in the range of 3.50 to 3.75, 3.75 to 4.0, and 3.75 to 4.0, respectively, were more likely to be accepted to medical school, a significant number of such applicants were not accepted. Again, these findings underscore the importance of a wide variety of personal characteristics and experiential variables in the medical student selection process.

Source: AAMC Data Warehouse: Applicant Matriculant File

As of October 15, 2014

MCAT and Undergraduate GPA

Chart 10-H combines MCAT scores and undergraduate GPA for all applicants to medical school from 2012 to 2014. The data may not reflect your particular circumstances. As a result, we recommend that you go to *www.aamc.org/facts* to see acceptance rates for particular demographic groups. Note that these results are presented without regard to any of the other selection factors.

Chart 10-H

MCAT® and GPA Grid, Applicants and Acceptees, 2012–2014 (aggregated)

GPA Total		MCAT® Total									
		3–14	15–17	18–20	21–23	24–26	27–29	30–32	33–35	36–38	39–45
3.8–4.00	Acceptees	3	4	57	317	1,363	4,232	7,110	6,298	3,688	1,385
	Applicants	80	162	524	1,526	3,554	6,978	9,361	7,504	4,176	1,519
	Accs/Apps	3.8	2.5	10.9	20.8	38.4	60.6	76.0	83.9	88.3	91.2
3.60–3.79	Acceptees	0	8	83	371	1,332	3,725	5,997	4,513	1,782	435
	Applicants	178	367	1,024	2,332	4,866	8,284	9,359	5,973	2,235	514
	Accs/Apps	0.0	2.2	8.1	15.9	27.4	45.0	64.1	75.6	79.7	84.6
3.40–3.59	Acceptees	1	13	67	314	1,010	2,307	3,600	2,382	819	176
	Applicants	337	553	1,278	2,607	4,691	7,151	7,455	3,854	1,176	234
	Accs/Apps	0.3	2.4	5.2	12.0	21.5	32.3	48.3	61.8	69.6	75.2
3.20–3.39	Acceptees	0	5	41	249	604	1,012	1,453	889	316	74
	Applicants	370	561	1,168	2,262	3,344	4,369	4,106	1,902	547	113
	Accs/Apps	0.0	0.9	3.5	11.0	18.1	23.2	35.4	46.7	57.8	65.5
3.00–3.19	Acceptees	0	2	25	123	373	455	530	313	112	21
	Applicants	388	553	928	1,578	2,218	2,361	1,851	808	233	40
	Accs/Apps	0.0	0.4	2.7	7.8	16.8	19.3	28.6	38.7	48.1	52.5
2.80–2.99	Acceptees	0	4	19	54	132	158	179	85	22	7
	Applicants	372	386	626	908	1,069	998	746	310	86	24
	Accs/Apps	0.0	1.0	3.0	5.9	12.3	15.8	24.0	27.4	25.6	29.2
2.60–2.79	Acceptees	0	1	12	24	47	57	59	33	15	3
	Applicants	275	284	355	486	512	388	276	117	47	10
	Accs/Apps	0.0	0.4	3.4	4.9	9.2	14.7	21.4	28.2	31.9	30.0
2.40–2.59	Acceptees	0	0	2	8	19	22	18	6	3	1
	Applicants	196	151	179	240	221	152	109	37	17	2
	Accs/Apps	0.0	0.0	1.1	3.3	8.6	14.5	16.5	16.2	17.6	50.0
2.20–2.39	Acceptees	0	0	0	0	7	8	6	1	0	0
	Applicants	132	77	94	91	88	68	39	14	5	3
	Accs/Apps	0.0	0.0	0.0	0.0	8.0	11.8	15.4	7.1	0.0	0.0
2.00–2.19	Acceptees	0	0	0	0	0	2	2	0	0	0
	Applicants	53	40	42	28	30	14	11	2	0	0
	Accs/Apps	0.0	0.0	0.0	0.0	0.0	14.3	18.2	0.0	--	--
0.99–1.99	Acceptees	0	0	0	0	0	0	0	0	0	0
	Applicants	45	9	11	12	8	6	3	0	0	0
	Accs/Apps	0.0	0.0	0.0	0.0	0.0	0.0	0.0	--	--	--

Percent Accepted = ◻ <25%   ◻ 25% – 49%   ◻ 50% – 74%   ◻ 75% – 100%

Source: AAMC Data Warehouse: Applicant Matriculant File

As of October 29, 2014

Chart 10-I

Undergraduate Major Distribution, All Applicants, 2010–2014

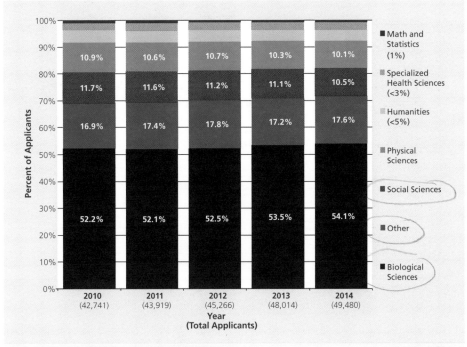

Source: AAMC Data Warehouse: Applicant Matriculant File

As of October 15, 2014

Chart 10-I presents information about the undergraduate majors of all medical school applicants to the 2010 to 2014 entering classes. Over the past five years, more than half of all applicants reported undergraduate biological science majors, while the remainder reported a variety of majors, including the humanities, mathematics and statistics, physical sciences, social sciences, other health sciences, and a broad "other" category. The proportion of these majors has remained relatively constant over time, despite annual fluctuations in the applicant pool.

Chart 10-J presents similar information about the undergraduate majors of applicants accepted to the 2010 to 2014 entering classes. Comparisons of the majors of the total applicant pool with those of accepted applicants reveal acceptance rates for various science-related majors ranging from 36.5 percent for applicants with specialized health science majors, to 42.2 percent for biological science majors, and to 49.4 percent for physical science majors, the highest rate of acceptance for science-related majors.

Chart 10-J

Undergraduate Major Distribution, Accepted Applicants, 2010–2014

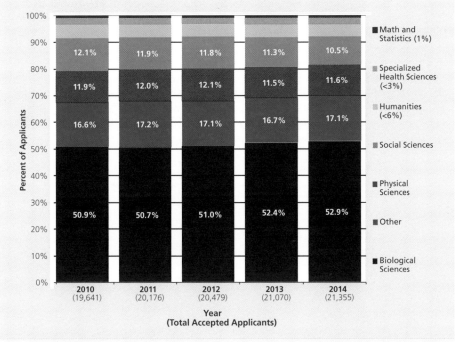

Source: AAMC Data Warehouse: Applicant Matriculant File

As of October 15, 2014

Gender

Chart 10-K presents information about the number and gender of the entire applicant pool and accepted applicants for the 1992 to 2014 entering classes. The largest annual applicant pool during the past 20 years was for the 2014 entering class, total for the 1996 entering class, which until 2013 was the largest applicant pool; after 1996, the pool gradually declined until 2003, when there was a slight increase (3.5 percent) in applicants. The applicant pool increased again by 2.7 percent in 2004, by 4.6 percent in both 2005 and 2006, and by 8.2 percent in 2007. In 2008 and 2009, the applicant pool held relatively steady, with a slight decrease of 0.2 percent from 2007 to 2008 and a slight increase of 0.1 percent from 2008 to 2009. In 2014, the applicant pool increased 3.1 percent from 2013. The number of male applicants to the 2014 entering class increased by 785 from the number of male applicants to the previous year's entering class, but that number was still smaller than it had been for each entering class from 1994 through 1996. The number of female applicants to the 2014 class increased by 769 over the number of female applicants to the previous year's entering class, the year 2014 having the largest number of female applicants on record. While the number of accepted applicants remained fairly constant for 10 years, it has started to increase in recent years, from a low of 17,312 in 1997 to a high of 21,355 in 2014. The number of accepted male applicants has fluctuated, from a low of 8,810 in 2003 to a high of 11,161 in 2014. The number of accepted female applicants has increased, with small fluctuations, from a low of 7,255 in

Chart 10-K

Applicants by Gender and Acceptance Status, 1992–2014

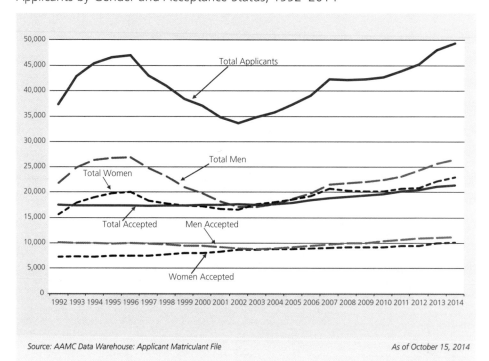

Source: AAMC Data Warehouse: Applicant Matriculant File

As of October 15, 2014

the 1994 entering class to a high of 10,194 in 2014. The significant gaps between male and female applicants for the 1992 entering class (6,166) and the 1993 entering class (6,892) have lessened; 553 and 301 more women than men applied to the 2003 and 2004 entering classes, respectively. In 2005, only 121 more men than women applied. In 2014, 3,436 more men than women applied to medical school. During the same time span, the gaps between accepted male and accepted female applicants also dropped. Accepted male applicants outnumbered accepted female applicants by 2,951 for the 1992 entering class, but only by 967 for the 2014 entering class. The national ratio of male to female applicants was 49.2 : 50.8 for the 2003 entering class, the first time that the number of female applicants to medical school was greater than the number of male applicants. For the 2004 entering class, this trend continued, with a ratio of male to female applicants of 49.6 : 50.4. For the 2005 entering class, there were once again more male than female applicants, with a ratio of male to female applicants of 50.2 : 49.8. This trend continued in 2014, with a ratio of male to female applicants of 53.5 : 46.5.

Chart 10-L

Age Distribution, Year 2014 Applicants

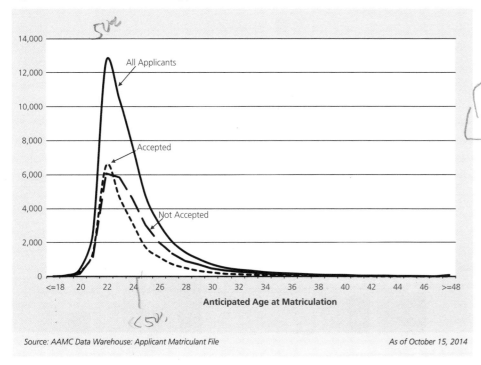

Source: AAMC Data Warehouse: Applicant Matriculant File

As of October 15, 2014

Chart 10-M

Percent of AMCAS® Applicants and Accepted Applicants Reporting Selected Experiences

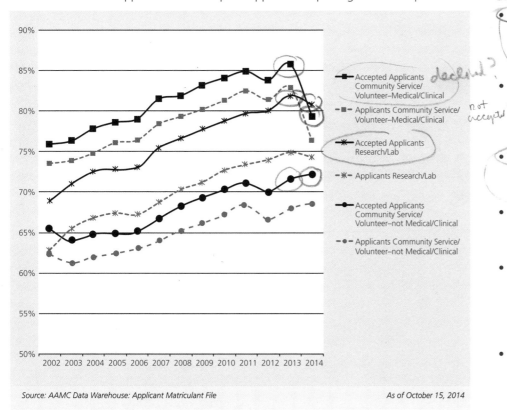

Source: AAMC Data Warehouse: Applicant Matriculant File

As of October 15, 2014

Age

Chart 10-L shows that the age distribution for all applicants to the 2014 entering class was broad, with 16 applicants under the age of 19 at the time of anticipated matriculation, and 81 applicants aged 48 and over. The largest contingent of applicants, 44,631, was between 21 and 28 at the time of anticipated matriculation; the rest of the applicant pool was either under 21 (502) or over 28 (4,347) at the time of anticipated matriculation. Chart 10-L illustrates a similar finding for accepted applicants. Accepted applicants for the 2014 entering class were between 17 and 58 years of age at the time of expected matriculation.

Applicant and Accepted Applicant Experiences

Chart 10-M presents information regarding the volunteer, paid, and lab experiences of AMCAS® applicants and accepted applicants to the 2014 entering class. The chart clearly shows the increase in both applicants and accepted applicants reporting volunteer medical, community service, and research experience since 2002:

- 79 percent of accepted applicants reported medical/clinical community service/volunteer clinical experience, an increase of about 3 percent since 2002.

- 76 percent of applicants reported medical/clinical community service/volunteer clinical experience, an increase of about 3 percent since 2002.

- 81 percent of accepted applicants reported research/lab experience, an increase of about 12 percent since 2002.

- 74 percent of applicants reported research/lab experience, an increase of about 12 percent since 2002.

- 72 percent of accepted applicants reported nonmedical/nonclinical community service/volunteer clinical experience, an increase of about 7 percent since 2002.

- 68 percent of applicants reported nonmedical/nonclinical community service/volunteer clinical experience, an increase of about 6 percent since 2002.

Self-Identity: All Applicants 2014

Chart 10-N shows applicant self-reported race and ethnicity data for all applicants from the 2013 and 2014 entering classes. Applicants can enter multiple races and ethnicities, so the sum of those shown does not equal the total number of applicants, nor are those for whom we have no race and ethnicity data included in this chart. Additional information for applicants from groups underrepresented in medicine is available in Chapter 8.

Chart 10-N

Distribution of Self Identity: All Applicants, 2014*

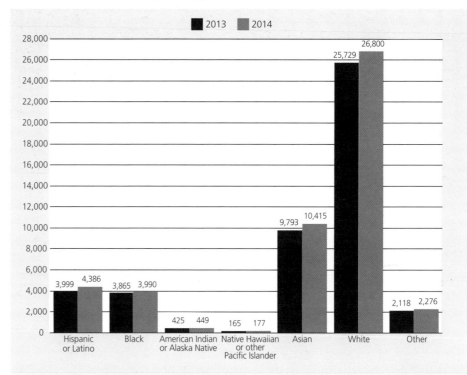

Source: AAMC Data Warehouse: Applicant Matriculant File

As of October 15, 2014

*Self Identities are reported for US Citizens/Permanent Residents only and may be alone or in combination with some other Self Identity.

Chapter 11:

You Can Afford Medical School

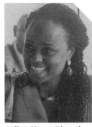

Juliet Siena Okoroh
Resident, General
Surgery
University of California,
San Francisco

There's no doubt that medical school is an expensive undertaking. Including the cost of tuition, fees, books, living expenses, and more, the average debt of a medical student in 2014 was slightly over $175,000.

The good news is that there are many tools and resources to help you manage your medical school expenses. After applying for financial aid, each medical school offers a financial aid package, which may include federal loans, program-specific scholarships for applicants with particular backgrounds and interests, and possibly grants. I chose my school because I felt like the faculty were really interested in me and made the best effort to offer me financial resources, which made it easy to concentrate on being a medical student without having to worry about how I was going to pay my rent.

With the average debt of medical students on the rise, it is very important to understand and discuss financial aid options. You should ask questions about the average debt of graduating medical students, but understand that everyone's situation is unique. So, be sure to consult with a financial aid officer or advisor before making any major decisions about how you'll manage your debt. Here are the personal debt management tips I've found helpful:

- *Develop a good relationship with your financial aid counselor or financial aid office.*

- *Create a reasonable budget.*

- *Live within your means and track your expenses.*

It's not always easy, but as you will learn in this chapter, there are various ways to finance your medical education. From grants and scholarships, to federal student loans, to service commitment programs that provide financial support, there are many resources available to help you navigate the process.

Distribution of Total Financial Aid

☐ Grants with a Service Commitment
■ Grants without a Service Commitment
▨ Loans

Source: 2013-2014 LCME Part I-B Student Financial Aid Questionnaire

Creating Your Budget

For assistance in creating a realistic budget, contact the financial aid office of the medical school you are interested in attending. Often they can provide some approximations on the average amount of student loan monies available to live on and the expected costs of necessities while a medical student.

Financial Information, Resources, Services, and Tools (FIRST)

FIRST is an AAMC program that provides a wide range of Financial Information, Resources, Services, and Tools to help medical school applicants and students make smart decisions about students loans, effectively manage their education debt, and expand their financial literacy skills.

Visit *www.aamc.org/first* for more information.

Building a Strong Financial Plan

You will need to develop a strategy to cover the significant costs associated with your education.

When you look at the figures in the table below, the financial challenges might seem overwhelming. Annual tuition, fees, and health insurance for the first year at state medical schools in 2014–2015 averaged approximately $33,107 and $56,730 for nonresidents; at private schools, the average was $52,046 and $53,653 for nonresidents.

Don't let these numbers discourage you. There's help available.

According to recent surveys conducted by the AAMC, 86 percent of newly graduated M.D.s have medical school education loans, while 61 percent reported receiving some degree of help through scholarships, stipends, and/or grants (which you don't have to repay). So, it can be done, and it is…by tens of thousands of medical students every single year.

But first… you will need a plan.

Before you can get to that crucial step of borrowing money, it's important that you understand—and adhere to—the basic principles of successful money management. With that in mind, the two basic recommendations that follow should help you build a strong financial foundation.

1) Live w/in your means
2) mng your debt wisely.

Table 11-A

Tuition, Fees, and Health Insurance for 2014–2015
First-Year Students in U.S. Medical Schools* (in Dollars)

Private Schools			
Student Category	**Range**	**Median**	**Average**
Resident	$20,665 - $61,436	$53,714	$52,046
Nonresident	$33,765 - $62,650	$55,044	$53,653

Public Schools			
Student Category	**Range**	**Median**	**Average**
Resident	$12,101 - $51,428	$34,540	$33,107
Nonresident	$22,113 - $86,403	$59,140	$56,730

*Analysis excludes East Carolina-Brody, Massachusetts, Mercer, Mississippi, and Southern Illinois. These schools do not accept nonresident medical students, and therefore, they do not report nonresident tuition and fees. Public medical schools excludes Uniformed Services University of Health Sciences, which does not charge tuition or student fees.

Source: 2013–2014 AAMC Tuition and Student Fees Questionnaire

Fixed vs. Variable Expenses

Categorize your expenses as "fixed" (ones that stay the same each month, such as rent and insurance premiums) or "variable" (such as groceries and clothing). This will help you identify areas in which you can scale back (if necessary) to ensure that your income and expenses remain in balance. Some easy cost-saving steps might be to share housing expenses with a roommate, buy generic products whenever possible, prepare more of your meals at home, and take public transportation or carpool.

Available Sources of Financing Include...

Grants, Scholarships, and Loan Repayment Programs
- Service Commitment Programs
- Scholarships for Disadvantaged Students
- Loan Repayment/Forgiveness Programs

Loans
- Direct Stafford Loans
- Direct PLUS Loans
- Federal Perkins Loans
- Primary Care Loans
- Loans for Disadvantaged Students

Information on these programs is provided on the following pages.

Overview: The Financial "Basics"

Live Within Your Means

All other efforts to "afford" medical school and handle your monies wisely will be undermined if you don't have a plan of action for your finances. Having a spending plan is the cornerstone of a solid financial foundation. Let's face it, money will be tight during medical school and a realistic spending plan will be critical to your financial well-being. A well-crafted plan will help you maintain better control of your spending, ensure you cover your essential expenses, and prepare you for unexpected expenses by building an emergency fund.

Creating a budget involves only a few steps:

- Income—document incoming funds, likely student loans, for the semester

- Expenses—identify the likely expenses for the semester

- Calculate—know the difference between income and expenses to see if you plan to live within your means.

Manage Your Debt Wisely

Given the costs of medical school, it's understandable that the vast majority of medical students borrow money to fund their education—and, as of 2014, graduate with median education debt of $180,000. Although the ability to manage debt wisely is important, regardless of one's situation, it becomes even more critical for you—a prospective medical student—when you consider the degree to which you're likely to rely on loans to help pay for your education.

- Be conscious of the amount you are likely to borrow and be comfortable knowing that your future income will be able to pay for your educational loan debt.

- Educate yourself on the various financing possibilities prior to arriving at medical school, but do not forget to also diligently search for free money like scholarships, grants, and repayment assistance programs.

- Understand that there are responsibilities, beyond making payments, that come with being a loan borrower. These include knowing what loans you hold, who to send payments to, and when payments are due. You will also be responsible for notifying your servicers of any changes to your name, contact information, or enrollment status.

- Stay organized. Maintain accurate financial aid records, copies of application forms, and any related paperwork. Of course, this also mean opening and reading all mail pertaining to your student loan debt. The Medloans® Organizer and Calculator is a tool that can help you keep everything documented. Every entering medical school student is given access to this resource, found at *www.aamc.org/first*.

- Build a good credit score by meeting your financial obligations. In doing so, you will strengthen your ability to qualify for and obtain attractive interest rates for credit-based loans, land a job, and rent an apartment. For more information, go to *www.aamc.org/first/creditscore*.

There are an abundance of resources to help you through this process—including those provided by your pre-health advisor, the pages that follow in this book, and the FIRST program offered by the AAMC. The financial aid package offered by each medical school may be a significant factor when it comes time to deciding which offer to accept. For information on this and other considerations, see Chapter 5, "Choosing the School That's Right for You."

Federal Student Loans for Medical Students

Characteristic	Primary Care Loan	Federal Perkins Loan	Direct Unsubsidized Loan	Direct PLUS Loan
Lender	Medical school financial aid office on behalf of the Department of HHS	Medical school financial aid office on behalf of the federal government	The federal government	The federal government
Based on Need	Yes[1]	Yes	No	No
Citizenship Requirement	U.S. citizen, U.S. national, or U.S. permanent resident	U.S. citizen, U.S. national, or U.S. permanent resident	U.S. citizen, U.S. national, or U.S. permanent resident	U.S. citizen, U.S. national, or U.S. permanent resident
Borrowing Limits	Up to cost of attendance (Third- and fourth-year students may receive additional funds to repay previous educational loans received while attending medical school)[2]	Up to $8,000/year, $60,000 cumulative (undergraduate and graduate combined)	$40,500 – $47,167/year, $224,000 cumulative maximum for premed and medical borrowing[2]	Annual cost of attendance minus other financial aid
Interest Rate	5%	5%	For loans disbursed after July 1, 2013, the rate is fixed for the life of the loan. These fixed rates are calculated every July 1st and are effective for loans disbursed during the next academic year. For current rates, visit http://studentaid.ed.gov/types/loans/interest-rates	For loans disbursed after July 1, 2013, the rate is fixed for the life of the loan. These fixed rates are calculated every July 1st and are effective for loans disbursed during the next academic year. For current rates, visit http://studentaid.ed.gov/types/loans/interest-rates
Interest Subsidy:	While in school, deferment, and grace period	While in school, deferment, and grace period	No	No
Grace Period	1 year	9 months	6 months	None
Deferments	While in school and during a primary care residency (check your promissory note or ask your financial aid officer)	While in school and other possible deferment periods based on eligibility (check your promissory note or ask your financial aid officer)	While in school and other possible deferment periods based on eligibility (check your promissory note or ask your financial aid officer)	While in school and 6 months after separating from school (post-enrollment deferment)
Repayment Requirements	Minimum: $40/month; 10 to 25 years to repay; Not eligible for loan consolidation	Minimum: $40/month, including interest; maximum 10 years to repay; eligible for loan consolidation	Repayment plans and postponement options exist during residency and beyond	Repayment plans and postponement options exist during residency and beyond
Prepayment Penalties	None			
Allowable Cancellations	Death or total and permanent disability			

[1] Borrower must agree upon signing loan agreement to enter and complete a primary care residency and practice in a primary care field, which together must be a total of 10-years in length or until the loan is repaid in full, whichever occurs first. Parent financial information is required for consideration for dependent students.

[2] Both annual and aggregate maximums are subject to change, pending congressional action.

Get Your Finances In Order

Before you apply for student loans, make sure your "financial house" is in order by:

- Creating a budget
- Paying down debt whenever possible
- Making sure you are current on all outstanding credit obligations

You Can Help Your Credit Score

- Pay your bills on time
- Limit your credit accounts
- Keep balances below your credit limit and pay off debt
- Check your credit report regularly at *www.annualcreditreport.com*

Students with a history of credit problems may not qualify for loans that are based on credit; this includes federal and private loans.

General Eligibility Criteria

Financial aid programs usually require that the applicant or student is:

- A U.S. citizen, or a permanent resident
- Making satisfactory academic progress
- Is in compliance with Selective Service registration requirements

Students With Medical School Loans

For the class of 2014, 84 percent of medical students graduated with education debt. The median amount of indebtedness for these graduates was $180,000. (This figure includes premedical school debt.)

Source: FIRST analysis of AAMC 2014 GQ Data

Students With Grants and/or Scholarships

61.4 percent of graduating medical students reported receiving financial assistance through grants, stipends, and/or scholarships in 2014. The average four-year total scholarship amount reported by those receiving scholarships was $60,059.

Source: AAMC's 2014 Graduation Questionnaire (GQ)

Types of Financial Aid

How will you pay for medical school?

First, remember that you're not alone. While the ultimate financial responsibility for your medical education rests with you and your family, there are many resources and tools available to help you. The financial aid officer at your medical school will assist you, but you will also want to talk to your pre-health advisor and familiarize yourself with the Financial Aid Fact Sheets on the AAMC FIRST website (*www.aamc.org/first*). Financial aid that typically is available to medical students includes loans, grants, and scholarships.

Loans

It is likely that your primary financial funding for medical school will come from federal student loans—a form of financial aid.

Federal loans are normally the first type of loan suggested, before considering private loans. The Loan Programs for Students table later in this chapter provides specific information about four of the most common federal loans used by medical students.

Medical school is expensive, but physicians' salaries are excellent. For example, the median starting salary for a family practice physician was $161,000*, and most other specialties have even higher starting salaries.

Make Sure You Are "Credit Ready"

Some medical schools require a credit history as part of the financial aid application and require that the applicant resolve any credit problems before the process gets underway. Some medical schools will grant a delay of matriculation to an accepted applicant who must address credit problems. Applicants are advised to contact financial aid offices at medical schools of interest to discuss financial aid eligibility and, if necessary, resolve any outstanding credit problems.

Grants and Scholarships

When it comes to financing your medical education, the best money is free money, often referred to as "gift aid," which you don't have to repay.

While grants and scholarships are likely to cover only a portion of your overall educational costs, it's worth noting that many students get some degree of funding from these sources. The source of gift aid can be from the federal government, the state government, other outside resources, and/or your medical school. Your medical school financial aid officer is the best source of information as to which grants and scholarships may be available to you.

The Financial Aid Application Process

The financial aid process may vary slightly by institution, so you will want to discuss each school's requirements with the financial aid officer. Regardless of the medical school, there's a standard process to apply for federal financial aid.

Step 1: Fill out the FAFSA

Completing the Free Application for Federal Student Aid (FAFSA) is the first step toward getting federal aid for medical school. Completing the FAFSA online is easy and free. It is best to submit the FAFSA form as early as possible in the calendar year—preferably after you've filed your income taxes—filling in both the student and parent

Per the MGMA Physician Placement Starting Salary Survey 2014 Report based on 2013 data.

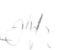

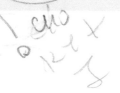

Service Commitment and Loan Forgiveness Programs

Learn more about these programs at the applicable website(s) listed below:

Army: www.goarmy.com/amedd/hpsp.html

Air Force: www.airforce.com/opportunities/healthcare/education

National Health Service Corps: www.nhsc.hrsa.gov/index.html

NHSC: Students to Service: http://www.nhsc.hrsa.gov/loanrepayment/studentstoserviceprogram/

NIH Loan Repayment: http://www.lrp.nih.gov/index.aspx

Navy: www.navy.com/careers/healthcare/physicians/

Public Service Programs: http://studentaid.ed.gov/repay-loans/forgiveness-cancellation/charts/public-service

State Programs: www.aamc.org/stloan

Education Tax Credits and Deductions

Education Tax Credits and Deductions
Do you know that the IRS can help you put some of the cost of medical school back in your pocket? It does so through (a) a student loan interest deduction of up to $2,500 for qualified individuals, and (b) the Lifetime Learning Tax Credit of up to $2,000 for eligible borrowers. ***Want to learn more? Read an overview of these programs—and learn the difference between a tax deduction and a tax credit. Click on "Education Tax Incentives" at*** www.aamc.org/first/factsheets.

---

information. The schools listed on your FAFSA will receive your financial information to then determine your eligibility for aid.

- **Step 2: Investigate Other Sources of Aid**
  Contact the financial aid office(s) at your medical school to investigate sources of institutional aid as well as learn about various student loan programs available.

- **Step 3: Receive and Reply to the Award Letter**
  Once your FAFSA and other required forms are received and processed by your medical school's financial aid office, you will receive an award letter indicating the types and amounts of financial aid for which you qualify—along with directions for accepting or declining the aid. For more information on award letters, review the Award Letter Fact Sheet: www.aamc.org/download/297592/data/awardletter.pdf.

The Federal Loans for Medical Students chart provides details on some frequently used federal loans in medical school, including Primary Care Loans, Federal Perkins Loans, Direct Unsubsidized Loans, and Direct PLUS Loans. For eligibility and additional details, talk with the financial aid officer at the medical school you plan to attend.

Financial Aid Principles When awarding aid, each financial aid office's principles are guided by multiple factors. The aid package is determined by available institutional resources, family resources, and the institution's mission. Additionally, the school compares the cost of attendance and other external variables before making a final determination of aid eligibility.

How Medical Schools Determine Eligibility for Financial Aid

Medical schools are sensitive to the financial needs of their students. Guided by federal regulations, the financial aid officer will determine your aid eligibility by examining the following principles:

- *How much does it cost?*
  The cost of medical education includes tuition, fees, books, supplies, equipment, and living expenses. These components make up the school's cost of attendance (COA) and vary by school. (You can find out the tuition and fees and COA of each medical school in the *Medical School Admission Requirements* website.)

- *What are your resources?*
  The next area that will be calculated is the amount you will be required to pay toward the cost of the education. This amount, called the expected family contribution (EFC), is determined through a need-analysis formula to ensure that all students are treated equitably. Both income and assets are considered.

  Even though you are considered to be independent for purposes of federal loans, many institutions require parental financial information to determine eligibility for institutional grants, scholarships, and school-based loans. School officials use this information to assess the student's ability to pay rather than willingness to pay, helping to ensure that certain types of aid are awarded to students with the greatest need.

- *What additional resources are needed?*
  Finally, the financial aid office will subtract your EFC from the institution's total cost of attendance. The remainder determines how much financial assistance you will require for the upcoming academic year. At this point, the medical school will then send you an "award letter" detailing the amount and type of financial aid available to you.

  You will be asked to accept or decline the offer (or a portion of it), and return the letter to the school. (The amount of financial aid an institution offers may be an important factor in choosing which school to attend. See Chapter 5 for additional information

---

and guidance on making your selection. To further assist you in the analysis of the awards letters, all accepted applicants are given complimentary access to the *Medloans Organizer and Calculator* [*www.aamc.org/first*]. This tool can be used to clearly see the total cost associated with the financing options provided in the award letters. You can choose the offer that appeals most to you.)

Forgiveness and Repayment Assistance Programs

There are loan forgiveness and repayment programs available for students interested in reducing their education loan debt through service. These are great options for those whose career goals align with those of the particular repayment/forgiveness program. The programs vary in structure, requirements, and award amounts.

The federal government provides both service commitment and loan repayment benefits to medical students interested in pursuing careers in primary care and those committed to working in a medically underserved area.

Additionally, the federal government has a program to reward borrowers of federal student loans who choose to work in public service with partial loan forgiveness. Student loan borrowers who choose certain repayment plans could also have portions of their debt forgiven if there is a balance remaining at the end of the term.

Individual state programs are available to students and graduates in return for a commitment to serve in the state's areas of need. Review the Loan Repayment/Forgiveness and Scholarship Programs database at *https://services.aamc.org/fed_loan_pub/index. cfm?fuseaction=public.welcome&CFID=7563505*.

The U.S. Armed Forces have programs that offer support to students enrolled in civilian medical schools in exchange for service in the branch that provided the funding.

For additional details on service commitment and loan forgiveness, please see the AAMC's FIRST Fact Sheets at www.aamc.org/first/factsheets, and for more detailed information about some of these programs, see the information on the following page.

Federal Loans and Repayment

There are a number of benefits available with the federal student loan programs. Some benefits include:

- Peace of mind. Payments are not required until after medical school is over. Payments can even be postponed throughout residency, if a borrower doesn't want to make payments during that time.

- Fixed interest rates. Rates will not rise and interest rate reductions may even be available if borrowers elect for automatic electronic payment and/or make their payments on time.

- Various repayment plans. Flexible plans are available to make payments affordable— even during residency.

As you near graduation, your financial aid office and your loan servicer(s) will provide you with the details you need to successfully manage your debt after graduation. To learn more, check out the FIRST Fact Sheets on loan repayment choices at www.aamc.org/first/ factsheets.

A Final Word About Financing Your Medical Education

The AAMC has a variety of financial information, resources, services, and tools for students and residents interested in learning about debt management. You are encouraged to use the resources at *www.aamc.org/first* to help you accomplish your financial goals. Best wishes as you embark on your pursuit of a career in medicine.

Chapter 12:

Information on Combined Undergraduate/M.D. Programs

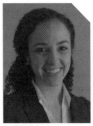

Stephanie K. Napolitano, M.P.H.
M.D. Candidate
Case Western Reserve University School of Medicine
Class of 2015

I was fortunate to attend a high school that emphasized the balance between academic rigor and a healthy personal life. This concept became very important to me, and I searched for the same balance when I applied to college. Knowing that I was interested in a future in medicine, I wondered if I would be able to find this balance as a premed student. I had seen family and friends struggle through the traditional medical school admissions process, and I knew it would be rigorous and challenging.

I learned about B.S./M.D. programs during a college interview. It sounded like the perfect way to achieve the balance I was looking for—a full four years of undergraduate studies (or a gap year if you finished your degree early), no required courses or major, the option to take either the MCAT® exam and apply elsewhere, or forego the stress and remain at the same university for medical school. I knew then that the B.S./M.D. program was for me.

If you're like me and you know you are dedicated to pursuing medicine as a high school student, the combined college/M.D. programs are an appealing opportunity. Programs range in length from six to nine years. During the initial two to four years, students complete their premedical coursework and earn their bachelor's degree. During the subsequent four years, students learn in a traditional medical school setting. These programs provide students with a wide variety of advantages, which may include a faster education track, freedom from application stress, and even liberation from the daunting MCAT exam. It's not for everyone, but if it's something you're considering, this chapter will give you a list of B.S./M.D. programs.

The purposes of these programs vary by institution, including:

- To permit highly qualified students to plan and complete a broad liberal arts education before initiating their medical studies

- To attract highly capable students to the sponsoring medical school

- To enhance diversity in the educational environment

- To reduce the total number of years required to complete the M.D. degree

- To educate physicians likely to practice in particular geographic areas or work with medically underserved populations

- To reduce the costs of a medical education

- To prepare physician scientists and future leaders in health policy

Potential applicants should familiarize themselves with the mission and goals statement of each combined degree program in which they have an interest to ensure a match between their educational and professional goals and those of the program.

These programs typically represent relationships between a medical school and one or more undergraduate colleges located in the same geographic region. They are sometimes part of the same university system, or they can be independent institutions.

Admission is open to highly qualified, mature high school students who are committed to a future career in medicine. Some of these programs are also open to college freshmen and sophomores. For more information, see the *Medical School Admission Requirements* website (*www.aamc.org/msar*), specifically the Application Requirements section for B.S./M.D. programs. State-supported schools generally admit few out-of-state applicants to their combined college/M.D. programs; private schools tend to have greater flexibility regarding state of residency.

While academic requirements vary among the schools sponsoring these programs, they typically include biology, chemistry, physics, English, mathematics, and social science courses. Calculus and foreign-language courses also are frequently required; a computer science course is sometimes recommended. Admission to the medical curriculum may occur immediately or after a student completes a prescribed number of semesters with a minimum grade point average (GPA). In some programs, students are not required to take the MCAT exam; in other programs, a minimum MCAT score must be attained for progression through the program.

Progressing through the program from the undergraduate to the medical curriculum is usually contingent on a student's achieving specific criteria in terms of standardized test scores, GPAs, and meeting the school's expectations regarding personal and professional behavior.

High school students interested in a combined undergraduate/M.D. program should consult their high school guidance counselor to ensure that they are enrolled in a challenging college preparatory curriculum, one that incorporates the specific courses required for admission to the program. The program descriptions in the *Medical School Admission Requirements* website were compiled from medical schools sponsoring programs of interest to high school students. For college freshmen and sophomores interested in these programs, please speak with your school's pre-health advisor. For additional information about specific programs, contact each school directly.

View complete, detailed information on each of the combined undergraduate/M.D. programs included in the two lists in this chapter, or in the *Medical School Admission Requirements* website.

MSAR Website Information

For more information about the *Medical School Admission Requirements* website, a preview of the site, and complete list of site features, data, and information, see *www.aamc.org/msar*.

List of Medical Schools Offering Combined Undergraduate/M.D. Programs by State, 2015–2016

Alabama

University of Alabama School of Medicine

University of South Alabama College of Medicine

California

University of California, San Diego, School of Medicine

Connecticut

University of Connecticut and University of Connecticut School of Medicine

Delaware

University of Delaware Medical Scholars Program

District of Columbia

The George Washington University School of Medicine and Health Sciences and The Columbian College of Arts and Sciences
Howard University College of Medicine

Florida

University of Florida College of Medicine

University of Miami Miller School of Medicine

Illinois

Northwestern University Feinberg School of Medicine

University of Illinois at Chicago College of Medicine

Massachusetts

Boston University School of Medicine

Michigan

Wayne State University School of Medicine

Missouri

Saint Louis University School of Medicine

University of Missouri—Kansas City School of Medicine

Nevada

University of Nevada

New Jersey

Rutgers New Jersey Medical School

Rutgers, Robert Wood Johnson Medical School

University of Medicine and Dentistry of New Jersey—New Jersey Medical School

New Mexico

University of New Mexico School of Medicine

New York

Brooklyn College and SUNY Downstate Medical Center

Hobart and William Smith Colleges/SUNY Upstate Medical University

Rensselaer Polytechnic Institute and Albany Medical College

St. Bonaventure University/The George Washington University School of Medicine and Health Sciences

Siena College and Albany Medical College

Sophie Davis School of Biomedical Education at the City College of New York

Stony Brook University and Stony Brook University School of Medicine

Union College and Albany Medical College

University of Rochester School of Medicine and Dentistry

Ohio

Case Western Reserve University School of Medicine

Northeast Ohio Medical University

University of Cincinnati College of Medicine

Pennsylvania

Drexel University and Drexel University College of Medicine

Lehigh University and Drexel University College of Medicine

Pennsylvania State University and Jefferson Medical College

Villanova University and Drexel University College of Medicine

Wilkes University/SUNY-Upstate Medical University

Rhode Island

Warren Alpert Medical School of Brown University

Tennessee

Fisk University and Meharry Medical College

Texas

Baylor University/Baylor College of Medicine (Baylor 2 Medical Track)
- Houston Premedical Academy
- Premedical Honors College (UT-Pan Am or PHC)
- Rice University and Baylor College of Medicine

University of Texas School of Medicine at San Antonio

Virginia

Eastern Virginia Medical School

Virginia Commonwealth University School of Medicine

List of Medical Schools Offering Combined Undergraduate/M.D. Programs by Number of Years, 2015–2016

6 Years
University of Missouri—Kansas City School of Medicine

6–7 Years
University of Miami

Northeast Ohio Medical University

Pennsylvania State University and Jefferson Medical College

7 Years
The George Washington University School of Medicine and Health Sciences and The Columbian School of Arts and Sciences

University of Florida College of Medicine

Northwestern University Feinberg School of Medicine

University of Illinois at Chicago College of Medicine

Boston University School of Medicine (8-year option available)

University of Medicine and Dentistry of New Jersey—New Jersey Medical School

Rensselaer Polytechnic Institute and Albany Medical College

Rutgers, Robert Wood Johnson Medical School

Sophie Davis School of Biomedical Education at the City College of New York

Drexel University and Drexel University College of Medicine

Lehigh University and Drexel University College of Medicine

Villanova University and Drexel University College of Medicine

Fisk University and Meharry Medical College

University of Texas School of Medicine at San Antonio

University of Nevada

8 Years
University of Alabama School of Medicine

University of South Alabama College of Medicine

University of California, San Diego School of Medicine

University of Connecticut and University of Connecticut School of Medicine

Howard University College of Medicine

University of New Mexico School of Medicine

Saint Louis University School of Medicine

Rutgers New Jersey Medical School

Rutgers, Robert Wood Johnson Medical School

Brooklyn College and SUNY Downstate Medical Center

Hobart and William Smith Colleges/SUNY Upstate Medical University

St. Bonaventure University/The George Washington University School of Medicine and Health Sciences

Siena College and Albany Medical College

Stony Brook University and Stony Brook University School of Medicine

Union College and Albany Medical College

University of Rochester School of Medicine and Dentistry

Case Western Reserve University School of Medicine

University of Cincinnati College of Medicine

Wilkes University/SUNY-Upstate Medical University

Warren Alpert Medical School of Brown University

Rice University and Baylor College of Medicine

Eastern Virginia Medical School

Virginia Commonwealth University School of Medicine

Wayne State University School of Medicine

University of Southern California College of Letters, Arts, & Sciences and Keck School of Medicine

Baylor University/Baylor College of Medicine (Baylor 2 Medical Track)

Houston Premedical Academy

Premedical Honors College (UT-Pan Am or PHC)

9 Years
University of Cincinnati College of Medicine (College of Engineering—undergraduate)

Chapter 13:

M.D.-Ph.D. Dual Degree Programs

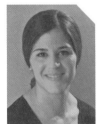

Catherine Spina
M.D.- Ph.D. Candidate
Boston University
School of Medicine
Class of 2015

As a science major in college, I developed an interest in research. I saw it as a way to actively engage in the process of discovery and innovation, ask new questions, and apply the technical knowledge I had been acquiring. I find becoming immersed in the question of how things work while generating and testing hypotheses about how to improve the pathophysiology of disease is extremely rewarding.

The rigor and intellectual stimulation of the research process engages and energizes me; however, I have been—and will always be—drawn to the bedside. The process of developing a connection with a patient, investigating his or her illness or disease, and offering relief for their suffering is immensely gratifying and meaningful.

Thus, in the laboratory, I have the potential to create, discover, and innovate with the long-term goal of impacting how we care for whole patient populations. While in the clinic, my impact as a physician is often immediate. Being unable to choose between science and medicine, I chose to pursue both through the M.D.-Ph.D. program. The combined degree program is the ideal training program for me because it supports my goal of translating basic research into clinical solutions and allows my clinical experience to inform and guide my research.

The Education of a Physician Scientist

Physician scientists—those who are trained in both medicine and research—are greatly needed in today's world. There is a synergy that results when experimental thinking and clinical practice are joined, and that combination is found among those who have completed both M.D. and Ph.D. degrees. These individuals help translate the achievements of basic research into active clinical practice and, in doing so, strengthen the link between medical knowledge and research as they prevent, diagnose, and treat disease. If this is the path you prefer, you will enjoy a busy, challenging, and rewarding career.

Advantages of the M.D.-Ph.D. Dual Degree

One route to a career as a physician scientist is enrollment in a combined M.D.-Ph.D. program. Although you can complete a Ph.D. program before or after receiving your M.D. degree, there are several advantages to pursuing joint M.D.-Ph.D. training:

- The greatest advantage of the dual degree program is the integration of research and clinical training. This integrated approach may include seminars that cross departments and interactions with teams composed of both basic science and clinical investigators.

- In addition, you can save a significant amount of time. Most M.D.-Ph.D. programs can be completed in a total of seven or eight years, compared to the nine or 10 it would take to earn both degrees independently.

- Students in M.D.-Ph.D. programs have access to opportunities for research and faculty mentoring to an extent frequently unavailable to M.D.-only students. As a result, these students are often able to enhance their mastery of the basic science background underlying patients' clinical problems and, ultimately, use that information to develop improvements in diagnosis and treatment.

Research Specialties

Just as with a Ph.D.-only career, students with a combined degree can pursue many scientific specialties. Most students earn their Ph.D. degrees in biomedical disciplines such as biochemistry, biomedical engineering, biophysics, cell biology, genetics, immunology, microbiology, neuroscience, and pharmacology.

It is important to realize that not every research specialty is offered at every medical school and that curricula can vary from institution to institution. In some schools, for example, M.D.-Ph.D. trainees also can complete their graduate work outside of laboratory disciplines in fields such as anthropology, computational biology, economics, engineering, health care policy, mathematics, physics, and sociology. View a summary of M.D.-Ph.D. programs and graduate fields of study at *https://www.aamc.org/students/download/62760/data/faqtable.pdf.*

Clinical Specialties

M.D.-Ph.D. students can pursue any one of many clinical specialties. The clinical specialty choices of students graduating from M.D.-Ph.D. programs over the past five years indicate strong interest in internal medicine, pathology, and pediatrics.

When compared to M.D.-only graduates, M.D.-Ph.D. graduates have been more likely to enter residencies in radiation oncology, child neurology, and pathology and are less likely to go into family medicine, emergency medicine, and obstetrics/gynecology. Additionally, the majority of dual degree students enter residencies after graduation. A small percentage of program graduates that do not enter residency typically go straight into a research postdoctoral fellowship position.

The Typical Program

Almost all U.S. and Canadian medical schools have M.D.-Ph.D. programs in one or more areas of specialization. (You can specifically search for M.D.-Ph.D. programs using the *Medical School Admission Requirements* website.) Some are relatively small in size (one or two new students each year, with a dozen or so total students), while others are much larger (up to 25 new students annually and a total enrollment of around 190).

Although there are differences among programs, core elements are common to almost all. The typical program is completed in a total of seven to nine years and includes:

- Completion of the first two years of combined medical and graduate school coursework

- Three to five years of doctoral research, including the completion of a thesis project

- A return to medical school for core clinical training and electives during the final years of the medical curriculum

At most schools, integrated approaches to graduate and medical education have been introduced throughout the curricula. In addition, most programs engage students in a wide

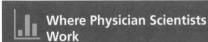
range of other activities to enrich their training experience. The median time for completion of a M.D.-Ph.D. program is eight years.

Residency Programs After Graduation

Several residencies around the country offer highly structured programs in which research is fully integrated into clinical training. They differ in their overall composition but generally offer a shortened residency training period. For more information, visit *www.aamc.org/students/research/mdphd/career_paths/.*

Application and Admission

Nearly all M.D.-Ph.D. programs participate in the American Medical College Application Service® (AMCAS®) application process described in Chapter 6.

If you choose to pursue the dual degree program, you will designate yourself as a combined M.D.-Ph.D. training applicant and complete two additional essays—one related to why you are interested in the joint training program, and the other describing your research experience. Specifics in the application process—and the prerequisites required for admission—vary from school to school. (Some institutions, for example, require GRE scores.) For complete information, make certain to review the description of the dual degree program at the website of each medical school in which you are interested.

Factors Considered by the Admissions Committee

Admissions committee members will review the application materials for the usual experiences, attributes, and metrics that are important for admitting students to M.D.-only programs (see Chapter 7). But because M.D.-Ph.D. applicants plan to become both physicians and scientists, committee members also will look for evidence of an applicant's passion and aptitude for research. They accomplish this largely through review of an applicant's statement of career goals and in letters of evaluation from faculty or researchers with whom the applicant has previously worked. In particular, committee members seek confirmation of:

- Relevant and substantive research experience during or after college

- An appreciation for and understanding of the work of physician scientists

- Intellectual drive, research ability, and perseverance

- Evidence of their passion and aptitude for research

If you hope to pursue the M.D.-Ph.D. joint degree, you will be expected to have clinical experience—either through volunteer work, shadowing a physician scientist, or specific training. Other experiences that admissions committee members look for are similar to those of the M.D.-only candidate, such as leadership positions, community service activities, and teaching roles.

Finally, it's important to be aware that while significant weight is placed upon an applicant's interest and experience in research activities, they are also expected to demonstrate a degree of academic excellence similar to those accepted in the M.D.-only program. For students entering M.D.-Ph.D. programs in 2014, for example, the mean GPA for students was 3.8 and total MCAT score was 35.0 as reported by AMCAS® *https://www.aamc.org/download/321548/data/2013factstable35.pdf.*

Keep in mind that the range of GPAs and MCAT scores for accepted applicants is quite broad and is considered in conjunction with other selection factors.

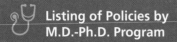

Listing of Policies by M.D.-Ph.D. Program

Review policies of M.D.-Ph.D. programs at *www.aamc.org/students/download/62760/ data/faqtable.pdf.*

Medical Scientist Training Program (MSTP)

The MSTP currently has 43 participating programs with a total of 932 trainees. About 170 positions for new students are available nationwide each year. For more information, visit *http://www.nigms.nih.gov/ Training/InstPredoc/Pages/PredocOverview- MSTP.aspx.*

Acceptance Policies

Just as application requirements vary from school to school, so do their acceptance policies. Some institutions permit an applicant who is not accepted to the M.D.-Ph.D. dual degree program to pursue admission to the M.D.-only curriculum. Other medical schools will accept applications from M.D.-Ph.D. candidates only for both degree programs, and failure to gain admittance to one program precludes consideration from another. Because school policies differ, applicants should clarify these matters at each school prior to applying and let admissions office staff know of their interest in pursuing an M.D.-only program (if that is the case) should they not be admitted to the dual degree program.

Financing M.D.-Ph.D. Programs

The sources of funding for M.D.-Ph.D. programs vary from school to school. Many schools offer full support for both the M.D. and Ph.D. components of their education, including tuition waivers, stipends, and health insurance. At other institutions, varying degrees of support are available, sometimes only for the Ph.D. component of the program. Before you apply to an M.D.-Ph.D. dual degree program, you should determine the level of financial assistance available.

A significant amount of funding comes from institutional sources and both individual and institutional grants. The latter includes the Medical Scientist Training Program (MSTP) sponsored by the National Institutes of Health (NIH), as well as other NIH grants. While you will undoubtedly want to review the list of medical schools participating in the MSTP (*www. nigms.nih.gov/Training/InstPredoc/PredocInst-MSTP.htm*), you also will want to contact the program officials at the institutions of interest and review their websites for full information.

Bear in mind that although most M.D.-Ph.D. programs offer support for their students, additional resources are available. Most take the form of competitive applications submitted by the trainee and their research mentor. These include fellowships from both private sources and a number of NIH institutes. You can review the list of these opportunities at *www.aamc.org/students/download/62756/data/fundingformdphd.pdf.*

For additional information and guidance about application to and enrollment in a combined M.D.-Ph.D. program, please visit the AAMC's website on the dual degree program at www. aamc.org/mdphd and contact your pre-health advisor and the M.D.-Ph.D. program director at the medical schools of interest.

For additional information regarding clinical specialties, see:

Brass LF, Akabas MH, Burnley LD, Engman DM, Wiley CA, Andersen OS. Are MDM.D.-PhD programs meeting their goals? An analysis of career choices made by graduates of 24 M.D.-Ph.D. programs. Acad Med. 2010; 85(4):692–701.

Paik JC, Howard G, Lorenz RG. Postgraduate choices of graduates from medical scientist training programs, 2004–2008. JAMA. 2009;302(12):1271–3.

Want to Learn More? You can find answers to questions frequently asked by students at: *https://www.aamc.org/students/research/mdphd/109850/mdphd_faqs.html.*

Chapter 14

Information About U.S. Medical Schools
Accredited by the Liaison Committee on Medical Education (LCME)

Medical School Admission Requirements Website—Complete U.S. Medical School Profiles

For complete, detailed information on each U.S. medical school, including MCAT® and GPA data, school-specific admission requirements and policies, applicant and acceptee statistics, and side-by-side medical school comparisons, purchase a subscription to the *Medical School Admission Requirements*. For more information about the *Medical School Admission Requirements* website, a preview of the site, and a complete list of site features, data, and information, visit *www.aamc.org/msar*.

U.S. Medical Schools

Alabama
University of Alabama School of Medicine

University of South Alabama College of Medicine

Arizona
University of Arizona College of Medicine - Phoenix

University of Arizona College of Medicine - Tucson

Arkansas
University of Arkansas College of Medicine

California
Keck School of Medicine of the University of Southern California

Loma Linda University School of Medicine

Stanford University School of Medicine

University of California, Davis, School of Medicine

University of California, Irvine, School of Medicine

University of California, Los Angeles, David Geffen School of Medicine at UCLA

University of California, Riverside, School of Medicine

University of California, San Diego, School of Medicine

University of California, San Francisco, School of Medicine

Colorado
University of Colorado School of Medicine

Connecticut
Frank H. Netter MD School of Medicine at Quinnipiac University

University of Connecticut School of Medicine

Yale School of Medicine

District of Columbia
The George Washington University School of Medicine and Health Sciences

Georgetown University School of Medicine

Howard University College of Medicine

Florida
Florida Atlantic University Charles E. Schmidt College of Medicine

Florida International University Herbert Wertheim College of Medicine

Florida State University College of Medicine

University of Central Florida College of Medicine

University of Florida College of Medicine

University of Miami Miller School of Medicine

University of South Florida Morsani College of Medicine

Georgia

Emory University School of Medicine

Medical College of Georgia at Georgia Regents University

Mercer University School of Medicine

Morehouse School of Medicine

Hawaii

University of Hawaii John A. Burns School of Medicine

Illinois

Loyola University Chicago Stritch School of Medicine

Northwestern University The Feinberg School of Medicine

Rosalind Franklin University of Medicine and Science Chicago Medical School

Rush Medical College of Rush University

Southern Illinois University School of Medicine

University of Chicago Division of the Biological Sciences, The Pritzker School of Medicine

University of Illinois at Chicago College of Medicine

Indiana

Indiana University School of Medicine

Iowa

University of Iowa Roy J. and Lucille A. Carver College of Medicine

Kansas

University of Kansas School of Medicine

Kentucky

University of Kentucky College of Medicine

University of Louisville School of Medicine

Louisiana

Louisiana State University School of Medicine in New Orleans

Louisiana State University Health Sciences Center School of Medicine in Shreveport

Tulane University School of Medicine

Maryland

Johns Hopkins University School of Medicine

Uniformed Services University of the Health Sciences F. Edward Hébert School of Medicine

University of Maryland School of Medicine

Massachusetts

Boston University School of Medicine

Harvard Medical School

Tufts University School of Medicine

University of Massachusetts Medical School

Michigan

Central Michigan University College of Medicine

Michigan State University College of Human Medicine

Oakland University William Beaumont School of Medicine

University of Michigan Medical School

Wayne State University School of Medicine

Western Michigan University School of Medicine

Minnesota

Mayo Medical School

University of Minnesota Medical School

Mississippi

University of Mississippi School of Medicine

Missouri

Saint Louis University School of Medicine

University of Missouri Columbia School of Medicine

University of Missouri — Kansas City School of Medicine

Washington University School of Medicine

Nebraska

Creighton University School of Medicine

University of Nebraska College of Medicine

Nevada

University of Nevada School of Medicine

New Hampshire

Geisel School of Medicine at Dartmouth

New Jersey

Cooper Medical School of Rowan University

Rutgers New Jersey Medical School

Rutgers, Robert Wood Johnson
Medical School

New Mexico

University of New Mexico School of Medicine

New York

Albany Medical College

Albert Einstein College of Medicine of
Yeshiva University

Columbia University College of Physicians
and Surgeons

Hofstra North Shore — LIJ School of
Medicine at Hofstra University

Icahn School of Medicine at Mount Sinai

New York Medical College

New York University School of Medicine

State University of New York Downstate
Medical Center College of Medicine

State University of New York Upstate
Medical Center College of Medicine

Stony Brook University School of Medicine

University at Buffalo School of Medicine and
Biomedical Sciences

University of Rochester School of Medicine
and Dentistry

Weill Cornell Medical College

North Carolina

The Brody School of Medicine at
East Carolina University

Duke University School of Medicine

University of North Carolina at Chapel Hill
School of Medicine

Wake Forest University School of Medicine
of Wake Forest Baptist Medical Center

North Dakota

University of North Dakota School of
Medicine and Health Sciences

Ohio

Case Western Reserve University
School of Medicine

Northeastern Ohio Medical University

The Ohio State University
College of Medicine

University of Cincinnati College of Medicine

The University of Toledo College of Medicine

Wright State University Boonshoft
School of Medicine

Oklahoma

University of Oklahoma College of Medicine

Oregon

Oregon Health & Science University
School of Medicine

Pennsylvania

The Commonwealth Medical College

Drexel University College of Medicine

Jefferson Medical College of Thomas
Jefferson University

Pennsylvania State University
College of Medicine

Raymond and Ruth Perelman School of
Medicine at the University of Pennsylvania

Temple University School of Medicine

University of Pittsburgh School of Medicine

Puerto Rico

Ponce School of Medicine

San Juan Bautista School of Medicine

Universidad Central del Caribe
School of Medicine

University of Puerto Rico School of Medicine

Rhode Island

The Warren Alpert Medical
School of Brown University

South Carolina

Medical University of South Carolina
College of Medicine

University of South Carolina
School of Medicine

University of South Carolina
School of Medicine—Greenville

South Dakota
University of South Dakota Sanford
School of Medicine

Tennessee
East Tennessee State University
James H. Quillen College of Medicine

Meharry Medical College
School of Medicine

University of Tennessee Health Science
Center College of Medicine

Vanderbilt University School of Medicine

Texas
Baylor College of Medicine

Texas Tech University Health Sciences
Center at El Paso — Paul L. Foster School
of Medicine

Texas A&M University System Health Science
Center College of Medicine

Texas Tech University Health Sciences Center
School of Medicine

University of Texas Medical Branch
at Galveston

University of Texas Medical
School at Houston

University of Texas
School of Medicine at San Antonio

University of Texas Southwestern
Medical Center at Dallas Southwestern
Medical School

Utah
University of Utah School of Medicine

Vermont
University of Vermont College of Medicine

Virginia
Eastern Virginia Medical School

University of Virginia School of Medicine

Virginia Commonwealth University
School of Medicine

Virginia Tech Carilion School of Medicine

Washington
University of Washington
School of Medicine

West Virginia
Marshall University Joan C. Edwards
School of Medicine

West Virginia University School of Medicine

Wisconsin
Medical College of Wisconsin

University of Wisconsin
School of Medicine and Public Health

Chapter 15:

Information About Canadian Medical Schools
Accredited by the LCME and by CACMS

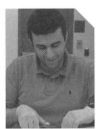

Basheer Elsolh
M.D.Candidate
Queen's University
School of Medicine
Class of 2017

Having completed my undergraduate education in Canada, I decided to pursue medical training there as well. As a result of having to meet the same LCME requirements as American programs, Canadian medical school curriculums are very similar to those taught in the United States. I particularly enjoy focusing on problem-based and simulation-based medical education, as it allows me to practice my skills and hone my knowledge in a risk-free educational setting. I chose Queen's University in particular because of the exceptional sense of collegiality that is prevalent in the faculty of medicine, as well as its focus on technological innovation in education and hands-on training through early clinical exposure.

Despite its large geographical dimensions, Canada only has 17 medical schools. Reflecting Canada's official bilingualism, 13 of these programs are exclusively English-speaking, three are exclusively French-speaking, and one is fully bilingual. Canadian medical schools are united under the Association of Faculties of Medicine of Canada (AFMC, www.afmc.ca), and all are affiliate members of the Association of American Medical Colleges (AAMC, www.aamc.org). All Canadian medical schools are officially accredited by both the U.S. Liaison Committee on Medical Education (LCME, www.lcme.org), and the Canadian Committee on Accreditation of Canadian Medical Schools (CACMS, www.afmc.ca/accreditation-cacms-e.php).

Selection Criteria

Canadian medical schools vary with respect to the number of years of undergraduate instruction required of applicants. Medical schools also vary with respect to the recommended content covered during premedical undergraduate education. Table 15-A shows that physics, inorganic and organic chemistry, biology, biochemistry, humanities, and English are the most common subjects required in undergraduate education by Canadian medical schools.

Language of Instruction

Three Canadian medical schools—Laval, Montréal, and Sherbrooke, all located in Quebec province—require students to be fluent in French as all instruction is in that language. Instruction in thirteen other schools is in English, and the University of Ottawa offers the M.D. curriculum in both French and English.

In Canada, universities fall under provincial jurisdiction and the majority of places in each faculty of medicine are allocated to permanent residents of the province in which the university is located.

Not all faculties of medicine accept applications from international students. Conversely, some faculties of medicine may reserve positions for international students, possibly as part of agreements with foreign governments and institutions. Statistics compiled by the

Table 15-A

Subjects Required by Two or More Canadian Medical Schools, 2014–2015 Entering Class

Required Subject	# of Schools
Biochemistry	4
Biology	6
Calculus	4
College English	2
College Mathematics	3
Humanities	2
Inorganic Chemistry	5
Organic Chemistry	7
Physics	5
Social Sciences	2

NOTE: n=17. Figures based on data provided fall 2013. Four of the 17 medical schools (Dalhousie, Northern Ontario, McMaster, and Western Ontario) did not indicate specific course requirements and are not included in the tabulations.

Association of Faculties of Medicine of Canada (*www.afmc.ca*) show that most medical schools admit international students. In 2013–2014, 83 U.S. students applied to 11 schools.

Canadian medical schools that supplied data recorded a 7.2 percent success rate. In the same year, 243 non-U.S. international students applied to the 11 Canadian medical schools that supplied data and recorded a 4.1 percent success rate. The success rate for Canadian applicants to the same schools was 22.5 percent. Additional information about Canadian medical schools can be found in the Association of Faculties of Medicine of Canada publication, Admission Requirements of Canadian Faculties of Medicine (2014) *www.afmc.ca/publications-admission-e.php*.

Positions filled by international students in Canadian medical schools are not necessarily subsidized by provincial/territorial governments. As such, international students, including U.S. students, may pay higher tuition and fees compared to those of Canadian residents.

Academic Record/Suitability

Although an excellent academic record is a very important factor in gaining admission to a Canadian medical school, admissions committees also put a great deal of effort into assessing applicants' suitability for a medical career based on other factors. Personal suitability is assessed differently by each school, but in general, personal qualities related to medicine are very important. Applicants who can demonstrate that they possess the qualities considered important in the practice of medicine may sometimes be admitted even if their academic record is not outstanding. Alternately, applicants with outstanding records who do not possess these qualities may not gain a place in medical school.

Most applicants to Canadian medical schools are interviewed prior to acceptance, so the interview information in Chapter 7 is relevant for applicants to Canadian medical schools as well.

Table 15-B

Tuition and Student Fees for 2014–2015 First-Year Students at Canadian Medical Schools (in Canadian Dollars)

Categories of Students	Range	Average
In-Province	$4,482 – $26,416	$15,503*
Canada, Out-of-Province	$7,521 – $26,416	$17,173*
Visa	$18,532 – $64,967	$33,461*

NOTE: Figures based on data provided Fall 2014

* Average in -Province data were derived from all 17 Canadian schools. Average Out-of-Province data were derived from all 17 Canadian schools. Average Visa data were derived from 7 schools that accept foreign students.

Source: Association of Faculties of Medicine of Canada

Medical College Admission Test® (MCAT®)

Twelve Canadian medical schools require applicants to take the MCAT exam: Alberta, British Columbia, Calgary, Dalhousie, Manitoba, McGill, McMaster, Memorial, Queen's, Saskatchewan, Toronto, and Western Ontario.

Other Considerations

Canadian faculties of medicine do not discriminate on the basis of race, religion, or gender in admitting new students. The admission of Aboriginal students (First Nations, Inuit, Métis) is encouraged at Canadian medical schools and most allocate positions specifically for Aboriginal applicants including Laval, Sherbrooke, Montréal, McGill, Ottawa, Queen's, McMaster, Western Ontario, Northern Ontario School of Medicine, Saskatchewan, Alberta, and British Columbia.

The number of female applicants has leveled off in recent years, with correspondingly consistent proportions of women in schools' entering classes. Women comprised 55 percent of the 2013–2014 applicant pool, and the success rate for women was slightly higher than that for men. The 2013 entering classes at the 11 Canadian medical schools reporting data about male and female matriculants included 55 percent women and 45 percent men. Overall, 22 percent of applicants received at least one offer of admission.

Expenses/Financial Aid

Tuition and student fees for Canadian and non-Canadian students in the 2013 entering class are provided in Table 15-B and in individual school entries. Expenses vary from school to school and from student to student. Tuition at several Canadian schools is slightly higher for the first year than for successive years. Some financial aid information is provided in the individual school entries. Eligible Canadian students may apply for a Canadian student loan, or they may apply to the Department of Education in their province for a provincial student loan.

Canadian Medical Schools

Alberta
University of Alberta Faculty of Medicine and Dentistry

University of Calgary, Cumming School of Medicine

British Columbia
University of British Columbia Faculty of Medicine

Manitoba
University of Manitoba Faculty of Medicine

Newfoundland
Memorial University of Newfoundland Faculty of Medicine

Nova Scotia
Dalhousie University Faculty of Medicine

Ontario
McMaster University, Michael G. DeGroote School of Medicine

Queen's University Faculty of Health Sciences

University of Ottawa Faculty of Medicine

University of Toronto Faculty of Medicine

Northern Ontario School of Medicine

Western University—Schulich School of Medicine & Dentistry

Quebec
Université Laval Faculty of Medicine

McGill University Faculty of Medicine

Université de Montréal Faculty of Medicine

Université de Sherbrooke Faculty of Medicine

Saskatchewan
University of Saskatchewan College of Medicine

Medical School Admission Requirements Website – Complete Medical School Profiles

For detailed information on each Canadian medical school, including MCAT and GPA data, school-specific admission requirements and policies, applicant and acceptee statistics, and side-by-side medical school comparisons, purchase the *Medical School Admission Requirements*. For more information about the *Medical School Admission Requirements* website, a preview of the site and complete list of site features, data, and information, visit *www.aamc.org/msar*.

Acronyms

AAMC
Association of American Medical Colleges
www.aamc.org

AMCAS
American Medical College Application Service®
www.aamc.org/amcas

FAP
Fee Assistance Program
www.aamc.org/students/applying/fap/

FIRST
Financial Information, Resources, Services, and Tools
www.aamc.org/first

MCAT
Medical College Admission Test®
www.aamc.org/mcat

Med-MAR
Medical Minority Applicant Registry
www.aamc.org/students/minorities/

SMDEP
Summer Medical and Dental Education Program
www.smdep.org

CiM
Careers in Medicine
www.aamc.org/cim

ERAS
Electronic Residency Application Service
www.aamc.org/eras

GHLO
Global Health Learning Opportunities
www.aamc.org/ghlo

VSAS
Visiting Student Application Service
www.aamc.org/vsas

FAFSA
Free Application for Federal Student Aid
https://fafsa.ed.gov/

NHSC
National Health Service Corps
http://nhsc.hrsa.gov/

NRMP
National Resident Matching Program
www.nrmp.org

USMLE
United States Medical Licensing Examination
http://www.usmle.org/

EDP
Early Decision Program

TSF
Tuition and Student Fees Sruvey

COA
Cost of Attendence

LCME
Liaison Committee on Medical Education
www.lcme.org

AFMC
Association of Faculties of Medicine of Canada
https://www.afmc.ca/

GQ
Graduation Questionnaire

MSQ
Matriculating Student Questionnaire

NAAHP
National Association of Advisors for the Health Professions
www.naahp.org

NBME
National Board of Medical Examiners
www.nbme.org/